WALK
FOR
HEALTH

THE NO NONSENSE LIBRARY

NO NONSENSE HEALTH GUIDES

Women's Health and Fitness
A Diet for Lifetime Health
A Guide to Exercise and Fitness Equipment
How to Tone and Trim Your Trouble Spots
Stretch for Health
Unstress Your Life
Calories, Carbohydrates and Sodium
Permanent Weight Loss
All about Vitamins and Minerals
Your Emotional Health and Well-Being
Reducing Cholesterol
Lower Your Blood Pressure
Soothe Your Aches and Pains
The Fiber Primer

NO NONSENSE FINANCIAL GUIDES

NO NONSENSE REAL ESTATE GUIDES

NO NONSENSE LEGAL GUIDES

NO NONSENSE CAREER GUIDES

NO NONSENSE SUCCESS GUIDES

NO NONSENSE COOKING GUIDES

NO NONSENSE WINE GUIDES

NO NONSENSE PARENTING GUIDES

NO NONSENSE STUDENT GUIDES

NO NONSENSE AUTOMOTIVE GUIDES

NO NONSENSE PHOTOGRAPHY GUIDES

NO NONSENSE GARDENING GUIDES

WALK FOR HEALTH

How to Start a Personal Fitness Program

By the Editors of *PREVENTION* Magazine

Longmeadow Press

Notice

This book is intended as a reference volume only, not as a medical manual or guide to self-treatment. It is not intended as a substitute for the medical advice of physicians. The reader should regularly consult a physician in general, and particularly for any symptoms. If you suspect that you have a medical problem, we urge you to seek competent medical help. Keep in mind that exercise and nutritional needs vary from person to person, depending on age, sex, health status, and other individual variations. The information here is intended to help you make informed decisions about your health, not as a substitute for any treatment that may have been prescribed by your doctor.

Library of Congress Cataloging-in-Publication Data

Walk for health : how to start a personal fitness program / by the editors of Prevention magazine.
        p.   cm. — (No nonsense health guide)
    ISBN 0–681–41020–5 paperback
    1. Walking—Health aspects.   2. Physical fitness.   I. Prevention (Emmaus, Pa.)   II. Series: No-nonsense health guide.
RA781.65.W34 1991
613.7' 176—dc20   80–2565
                                                                                      CIP

Compiled and edited by Marcia Holman

Book design by Rodale Design Staff

Photographs by Angelo Caggiano, pp. 3, 64; John P. Hamel, p. 18; Rodale Stock Images, pp. 33, 42; Sally Shenk Ullman, pp. 49, 58, 81.

Printed in the United States of America on acid-free paper

0 9 8 7 6 5 4 3   paperback

Contents

This funny-looking style of walking has serious health
benefits—it whittles your waist, slims your hips, and
tones you all over.

Busy schedule? Foul weather? Inspirational tips to
help you stay motivated and stick with your fitness
walking program.

Walk Your Way to Total Health

Here's a prescription for nearly everyone, sick or well: Start a regular walking program and stay with it.

Walking regularly can help you shed weight, boost your energy, lower your blood pressure, relieve the pain of arthritis, promote lung health, and alleviate mental depression as well as reverse bone loss that so often accompanies aging.

That might seem like a pretty tall order for an exercise as easy as walking, but the health benefits of walking are backed by scientists who are finding that the world's oldest form of aerobic exercise may indeed be the best—one that could give you a new lease on life.

Let's take a look at the way walking whittles off weight, for example. Studies have shown that regular walking is better than dieting for reducing weight and keeping it off. The reason? Walking revs up your metabolism which means it burns calories (about 100 per mile for a 150-pound person), and it keeps burning them at a faster-than-normal pace for several hours after, even if all you do is stretch out on the couch.

Besides burning fat, walking builds muscle, and muscle tissue burns calories even faster than fat does!

While walking is trimming your body, it also helps tune up your heart. Studies have shown that a regular walking program boosts levels of HDL or high-density lipoprotein—the good kind of cholesterol that protects against heart disease. At the same time, walking decreases artery-clogging blood fats and prevents blood clots that could lead to a heart attack. And that's not all. Walking has been found to lower blood pressure even more effectively than drugs for some people.

As if strengthening your heart and keeping you trim weren't enough, walking can also stop the progression of varicose veins, ease your headaches, and help your muscles take up blood sugar, which can prevent or alleviate diabetes. Furthermore, walking helps bones take on more calcium and become thicker and more resistant to osteoporosis.

Walking is also a great tonic for your mind. When you're striding along, with your arms swinging and your head held high, stress and worry just seem to dissolve away. The reason, say scientists, may be that walking helps release endorphins, your body's natural mood-elevating chemicals.

The ease of walking is the secret to its advantages. It gives you the benefits of more strenuous forms of exericse—but without the beating. Much more important than distance or speed is regularity. Walking day after day, month after month, is what seems to produce the best health results.

Start taking your walking prescription today. If you stick with it, you may not need another prescription for a long, long time.

Walk for Health will help get you started on your lifetime walking program. You'll learn how to use walking to lose weight, prevent heart disease, control diabetes, and manage stress. You'll also learn how to prepare your body for fitness walking, which shoes to wear, and, most important, how to pace yourself so that you can gradually work your way toward more energetic walking. Finally, you'll find lots of inspiring ways to keep you walking every day—even when your schedule is full and the weather is foul.

CHAPTER
ONE

On the Road
to Permanent
Weight Loss

Scientists are impressed, and walkers are delighted: Unwanted pounds are coming off, and staying off for good, to the steady beat of walking feet.

But why? What makes walking so tough on unwanted pudge?

As obesity experts point out, one of the most common pitfalls of starting an exercise program is trying to do too much too soon. "Many people have an all-or-nothing attitude about exercise," points out bariatric physician Scott Rigden, M.D., of Tempe, Arizona. But walking offers a wide range of acceptable paces—from a slow stroll for beginners to a brisk arm-pumping stride later on.

Walking burns calories at any speed. Of course, brisker walking burns more. But if you can't (or don't want to) go faster, you can walk longer to make up the difference. For example, if you weigh 150 pounds and cover 1 mile in 15 minutes (that's 4 mph), you burn about 110 calories. But walk at a slower pace (3 mph) and you get the same calorie burn in just 1 1/10 mile. "This is truly a race that the tortoise wins, not the hare," says cardiologist James

Rippe, M.D., director of the exercise physiology laboratory at University of Massachusetts Medical Center in Worcester.

In many ways, walking may be even better than jogging if you have more than a few pounds to lose. True jogging burns about 20 percent more calories than brisk walking. But compare how you feel at the end of a 3-mile walk with how you feel when you jog that same distance. Jogging may take more out of you if you're overweight. With less chance of injury and fatigue, even out-of-shape people can exercise longer and more frequently by walking. In reality, that translates into a greater number of calories burned.

So if you want to win the battle of the bulge, you don't have to become a marathon runner. We now have fresh evidence that an easy-to-moderate walk for less than an hour several times a week is all it takes to help you shed unwanted pounds and—best of all—prevent them from piling back on.

To find out why walking may be your best—and only—diet aid, read on.

How Walking Supercharges Your "Engine"

It's a fact that walking helps you burn calories while you walk and for a while after your walk is over. But here's even better news: This short "afterburn" can, in a sense, turn into a continual burn.

That's because walking regularly signals the muscle cells to increase the size and number of *mitochondria*—the structures that help burn calories as engines burn gasoline. Simply put, lean muscle burns more calories than fat ones do—an estimated 10 calories more.

It's as if walking fiddles with your body's carburetor. For up to several hours after you stop walking, your body's normal rate of burning calories gets stuck in a fast idle, revving at a higher rate than before you walked. Faster burn means faster weight loss. So the more you walk, the faster your fuel guzzling.

Walking uses more fat for energy.   Walking increases the concentration of oxidative enzymes in your cells. These en-

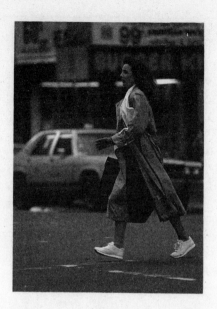

If you want to lose weight, use footpower to get around. The average-size person walking at an easy-to-moderate pace can burn about 100 calories a mile. If you walk three miles per hour, you could burn up to 300 calories an hour. Walk every day and you could lose two pounds a month—without cutting calories!

zymes are needed for fat metabolism. "Exercising improves the body's ability to use body fat for fuel," says Herman M. Frankel, M.D., national chairman of the Obesity Foundation and director of the Portland Health Institute, Portland, Oregon.

Walking helps you build lean muscle.   Walkers employ the so-called slow-twitch, rather than fast-twitch, muscles. A bird that flies over the Atlantic Ocean has slow-twitch muscles in its wings. Your legs have them, too. And guess what? The mitochondria in slow-twitch muscle fibers prefer to burn fat for fuel. "Muscles designed to do long, continuous movements tend to be the fat-burning type of muscle," says Peter D. Wood, Ph.D., professor of medicine, Stanford University Medical School, and associate director, Stanford Center for Research in Disease Prevention, Palo Alto, California.

Walking Sculpts Your Body

Walking not only helps you drop pounds but also whittles a leaner profile.

Look trimmer all over.   You'd probably expect walking to trim and tone your legs. And it does. But the flab trimming may not stop there. A study at the University of California reported "a striking loss of fat over the arm" in both walkers and cyclists after six months of regular exercise. Walking can take off fat anywhere—from jelly belly to thunder thighs.

Walking is an aerobic activity, which means it burns off body fat. And usually the areas of highest fat concentration melt away first. In men, that usually means the gut; in women, the hips and thighs. And, as we said, the good news is that you can burn off much of that fat!

"It won't all go away overnight. And some people won't take off as much as they'd like to in certain areas," explains Charles Eichenberg, Ph.D., director of the New Start Health Center, in St. Petersburg, Florida. "But for most of us, regular walking will make visible changes."

Tone all your muscles.   The sculpting effect isn't all due to fat loss. Walking tones up muscles, too—and, once again, the legs aren't the only beneficiaries. "Walking is a carefully designed balancing act. The muscles of the abdomen and lower back can receive a moderate workout just keeping your trunk in line with your legs during a brisk walk. That's how you keep moving forward without falling flat on your face," says Randall L. Braddom, M.D., director of physical medicine and rehabilitation at Providence Hospital, in Cincinnati.

Get an upper-body workout, too.   Your arms and upper torso also get a mild-to-moderate workout when you walk, because you naturally swing your arms. You can increase that workout by deliberately pumping your arms or by using hand-held weights.

Walking Is Better Than Dieting

Perhaps you've tried dieting or quick weight-loss remedies only to discover that, after a while, the pudge just doesn't budge, no matter how little you eat. Or maybe you've found that as soon as you lose, the weight creeps back on, pound by pound.

The reason this happens is that stringent dieting lowers the body's metabolism, which means that proportionately fewer calories are burned. Add an exercise like walking, however, and your excess baggage will melt off—and stay off.

There have been many studies showing that exercise is more effective than dieting for losing weight. In one, Grant Gwinup, M.D., professor of medicine and chief of the Division of Endocrinology and Metabolism, University of California, Irvine Medical Center, Orange, California, assembled a group of obese people who had all failed to lose weight by dieting. Dr. Gwinup asked them to continue their normal eating habits but to walk at least 30 minutes or more per day for a year. At the end of a year, all of the subjects had lost weight, at an average of 22 pounds each.

The best part about all this is that walking allows you to lose weight by increasing the number of calories you burn without decreasing your calorie intake. Perhaps if more overweight people thought of themselves not as overeaters but as underexercisers, there'd be a lot more slim and trim people in the world.

Take a 45-minute walk four times a week, for example, and you could drop almost 18 pounds in a year.

Walking keeps your appetite in check.   Contrary to popular belief, exercising does not necessarily make you work up an appetite. Scientists found this out by counting the calories consumed by a group of obese women during a two-month experiment. Each underwent three 19-day treatments—a sedentary period, a period of mild daily exercise, and a period of moderate exercise. Each woman was allowed to eat as much as she wanted, and although all of them gradually became more active, their caloric intake did not increase. Some experiments suggest that exercise may even help suppress appetite.

Walking stamps out stress eating.   Many people put on extra pounds by using food to deal with stress and tension. A bowl of ice cream subs as a tranquilizer. But while high-fat goodies travel straight to your hips and set up house there, a walk takes you way beyond the tension of the moment.

In a study at the University of Massachusetts Center for Health and Fitness, researchers found that walking reduces anxiety, no matter how casual or intense the workout. And this calming effect lasts for at least 2 hours after exercise.

How to Walk Your Weight Away

The strongest part of the human body is the legs. The weakest: that nodule of the brain in charge of resisting cookies. Therein lies the first secret of successful weight control. Through walking, what we do is substitute walkpower for willpower.

But just how much walking do you need to do for weight loss?

Regularity is more important than pace.   The walking prescription for weight loss is more immediately concerned with the number of calories burned during exercise than in the aerobic fitness, although ideally the two eventually go hand in hand. For that reason, it's less crucial to keep up the pace and more important to make sure that you meet a goal of, say, 3 to 5 miles on a daily basis. Even if you can only manage a half mile to start, walking every day gets you in the habit.

You can cover a mile in 15 to 20 minutes.   If you don't know how far you're walking, it's a good idea to use your car to measure off the mile markers on your favorite walking course. Failing that, figure that with brisk walking you generally cover 1 mile every 15 minutes. With what might be called easy-to-moderate walking you cover 1 mile in about 20 minutes.

How walking adds up to pounds lost.   Let's say you walk at an easy-to-moderate pace for 45 minutes. You'd be covering a little more than 2 miles (based on 20 minutes of easy-to-moderate-walking equals 1 mile). If you weigh 140 pounds, for instance, that's 95 calories you'd be burning per mile. So your total calorie burn for the walk would be 2 times 95, or 190, plus 25 calories for the "little more" equals 215 calories. Do that every day for 30 days, and you've walked away 30 times 215 calories or 6,450 calories. And what does that equal? Figuring that 3,500 calories equal 1 pound, you will have lost close to 2 pounds, which adds up to 22 fewer pounds of body fat after a year.

Another example: You walk an hour a day (maybe in two segments) at the same easy pace. That's 3 miles a day. If you weigh 170 pounds, that's good for 330 calories per day. Maybe you average six days a week (instead of seven as in the first example). Total calorie burn for a week: 2,010 calories. Multiply that by 52 weeks a year, and it equals 104,520 calories. Divide by 3,500 and you get a total weight loss of almost 30 pounds.

Calorie expenditures vary.   Keep in mind that these calorie expenditures are simply estimates. The actual number of calories you expend will vary slightly according to the distance you walk, your pace, your weight, how much clothing you wear, the terrain (hilly or flat), and even headwinds. If the terrain is hilly or you walk fast, for example, you'll burn more calories than if you stroll along on a flat terrain at a leisurely pace.

A simple equation for calories burned.   If you want to simplify matters, figure that if you walk at the leisurely pace of 3 miles per hour (1 mile every 20 minutes), you burn up to 300 calories an hour. Do that every day, and you can lose 2 pounds per month with no change in diet. Combine that with a 300-calorie-per-day cut in food intake, and you can drop 4 pounds per month!

If you move at a brisker pace of 4 miles per hour, you'll burn about 400 to 500 calories per hour.

Get into the Proper Mindset

Where walking is concerned, psychology is more important than math. As you may have gathered from the figures given, weight loss by walking is something that can be measured meaningfully over a period of months, not days. But don't let that discourage you. Tell yourself these facts, over and over again.

- I'm better off losing weight slowly. The more gradual the weight loss, the more likely it is to be permanent.
- By losing gradually, I'm preventing the baggy skin that could result if I lost more rapidly.
- This is the healthiest way to trim down. I don't have to cut back on good nutrition. I don't need diet pills.

Calories Expended to Walk 1 Mile

You don't have to be a math wizard to calculate how many calories are burned up when you walk. Simply figure that walking 1 mile will burn up approximately 100 calories. Or if you walk 1 mile and are in one of the following weight categories, you can burn up the following number of calories.

Approximate Weight	Calories Burned
120	80
130	85
140	95
150	100
160	105
170	110
180	115
190	120
200	125

And all the weight I'm losing is fat. (People who lose weight by dieting lose lots of muscle tissue as well as fat.) Even though I'm losing weight more slowly than a strict dieter, I'm ahead of the game!

These few final tips will help assure weight loss through walking.

Don't use walking as an excuse to eat carelessly.   Remember, the losses we're talking about will occur if you keep eating your normal diet. If you eat more than you usually do, you'll lose more slowly. Be aware of what you eat, when you eat, and why you eat.

Quench your thirst with low-cal drinks.   Drink plenty of water throughout the day.

Schedule your walk for the same time each day.   Stick to that schedule until it becomes a part of your life. Many people find that going to bed an hour earlier than usual and then walking during the fresh dawn hours is the best solution.

Wear a good pair of walking shoes.   If you're more than 20 pounds overweight and you've been inactive for a while, make a point to get good-quality walking shoes before you start exercising. Good shoes are important for all exercise walkers, but even more so for inactive people with a lot of weight to lose. People carrying a lot of excess weight are more prone to overuse injuries, such as plantar fasciitis (a common cause of heel pain), and general circulation problems in the legs and feet. Look for good arch support and plenty of toe room. (For more details on proper footwear for walking, see chapter 6.)

Get a medical checkup.   If you're 50 or more pounds overweight, seek a doctor's advice before beginning any exercise program, even walking. If you get chest pains during exercise or have chronic foot or leg problems, consult your personal physician.

Don't expect too much at first.   Keep your expectations in pace with your workouts. "If it took 40 years to get the body shape you have today, you can't expect to reverse the process in 40 days," says James Stray-Gundersen, M.D., assistant professor of surgery and physiology at the University of Texas Southwestern Medical Center. "Nature does things best gradually."

Keep on Walking!

Sometimes it can take a little extra effort to keep walking on the road to weight loss—especially if you're lugging around a spare tire or two.

Joe Owens, Ph.D., professor of exercise physiology and director of the fitness laboratory at the State University of New York at New Paltz, has been in the fitness business for more than 30 years. A former coach and athletic director and consultant, he's come up with plenty of tips for staying motivated. Here are eight encouraging tips from Coach Owens.

Make a list and check it twice.   Try to think of as many reasons as you can for maintaining a regular walking program. Your list might read like this:

"I can wear designer jeans. I'll perform better. I'll sleep better, eat better, get off some medication, eat more of the things that I like, feel more psychologically balanced, do better at work." Keep going!

Then, make a list of the reasons why you can't get out and walk regularly. That list will probably be a lot harder to compile!

Then compare your lists. The good things you achieve will far outnumber the reasons for not doing the walking. "I like to challenge people who want to lose weight to give me ten reasons why they can't without repeating themselves," says Dr. Owens. "They can't do it!"

Have a specific goal.   Create goals that allow you to achieve a little bit every day or every week.

Plan to walk a certain amount every day, based on your ability. Each day you achieve your goal, give yourself a mental pat on the back.

Visualize your goal.   Being able to see, feel, hear, and taste your goal is a powerful force in reaching it. Olympians imagine the roar of the crowds. The applause. The feeling of the gold medal being placed around the neck. They use all their senses to visualize their goal to keep motivation high.

You can do the same thing. Feel what it would be like to be walking at a brisk pace on a cool morning. Imagine what you'll feel like when you've achieved your weight-loss goal and you're still out there walking to maintain it. Imagine how much healthier you'll feel, how much easier your body will move, how the strength in your muscles will power you along, and how much easier your breathing will be. Feel the new energy your walking program will bring you.

Find a role model.   Find a person whom you'd like to emulate, a person who walks regularly and maintains his or her weight. What are his or her strategies for getting out there every day and walking? Take your cue from there. Identifying with a positive role model can be a real shortcut to success.

Be your own cheerleader.   If you miss a day, don't berate yourself. Give yourself encouragement even when you walk less than your goal. Tell yourself you have a goal, but that you're going to enjoy the battle even more than the victory. Then, get going!

Keep filling in your daily walking log.   Keeping a daily diary of when you walked, how far, and how you felt can be a great inspirational tool. (For more information on how to keep a walking log, see chapter 8.)

Add Hand Weights and Burn More

If you are in good health and want to burn even more calories, and also increase your level of aerobic fitness in the process, try carrying hand weights.

"Use hand weights during walking and you can burn more calories per mile than you would while running," says Bryant Stamford, Ph.D., director of the Exercise Physiology Laboratory at the University of Louisville School of Medicine.

A 150-pound man, for instance, could lose 126 calories a mile while walking 3 miles per hour, or 134 calories a mile when walking 4 miles per hour, if he carried 5-pound weights. Yet if he foregoes hand weights and runs at a pace of 6 mile per hour, he'll burn only 120 calories each mile.

If you opt for hand weights, Dr. Stamford offers the following advice.

Start light.   Start off with 2- or 3-pound weights and gradually work up to heavier weights.

Bend your arms.   Carry the weights with your arms bent and swinging. "Arm movements must be controlled because you can damage delicate elbow and shoulder tissues if the weights swing about indiscriminately," says Dr. Stamford. Carrying weights at your sides accomplishes little, because the weights aren't used actively in the walk. Ankle weights aren't recommended because they affect foot placement and walking style, which could lead to injuries.

A weighted belt works well, too.   Wearing a weighted

belt or vest may be superior to hand weights for some people since they are less likely to alter your stride and cause you to injure your arms or shoulders.

Here are a few additional ways you can boost your calorie loss while walking.

Walk on loose terrain.   Walking in sand or freshly plowed earth can boost calorie burn by an average of 30 percent, according to E.C. Frederick, Ph.D., of the Penn State Center for Locomotion Studies, and coauthor of *Walk On, a Tool Kit for Building Your Own Walking Fitness Program.*

Walk uphill.   At a pace of 4 miles per hour, if you walk up a 5 percent grade—a hill that'll rise about 5 feet for every 100 feet you cover—you'll burn about 45 percent more calories than while walking on a flat surface.

Small hills are best.   Naturally, the steeper the grade, the more calories you'll burn. But don't try walking up any pyramids at first. "Walking up grades is more strenuous than normal flat-land walking, and it strains your entire body, especially your cardiovascular system," says Dr. Frederick. "A 5 or 10 percent grade should cause no problem, but a person should be in good shape to tackle anything steeper." (For perspective, consider that a 5 percent incline is about the steepest grade on a freeway, and stairs are about a 50 percent grade.)

Walk farther, walk faster.   Every extra mile can smoke off another 100 calories. If you're pressed for time, gradually get accustomed to walking a little faster.

How to Fight Heart Disease and Catch Up to Good Health

Ralph Riemer, 45, was working as a respiratory equipment technician at St. Mary's Hospital in Rochester, Minnesota, when he began to have chest pains. He'd had similar symptoms for a few weeks each time he walked up a long ramp at the hospital. This time, though, the pain didn't disappear when he sat down to rest; his arm and neck started to ache, too. Riemer headed for the emergency room, where his fears were confirmed: He was having a heart attack.

Tests revealed that Riemer had two blocked arteries. Both were opened with an operation called balloon angioplasty. Then, at his doctor's behest, Riemer began doing something he'd been postponing for years: He started to exercise.

Within days of his heart attack, he was given an exercise (treadmill) stress test. A week later he started working out on a treadmill at a nearby cardiac rehabilitation center. From there, he started walking around his neighborhood. At first he put in about a mile a day. Eventually he worked up to five miles a day, at least three times a week.

The results of his walking program were nearly astonishing. Riemer lost 30 pounds; his cholesterol fell into the safe range; his resting pulse rate dropped 30 points. "It's nice to have a second chance," he says. "I haven't felt this good in years."

Indeed, studies show that walking can make your heart beat as if you were years younger.

The best news of all is this: A strengthened heart can mean a longer life. In one major study, some 12,000 men who were at risk for developing heart disease were followed over a seven-year period. During the follow-up, researchers at the University of Minnesota School of Public Health found that those men who were moderately active in their leisure time had 30 percent fewer deaths from heart attacks than more sedentary men.

What's just as impressive is the evidence that shows that even if you have a heart condition and have had a heart attack, an exercise like walking can actually reverse the damage and prevent you from having a second heart attack. Canadian researchers studied more than 600 post-coronary patients who exercised regularly and compared them to heart patients who didn't exercise. Their finding? The patients who exercised were nearly five times less likely to suffer a second heart attack.

Walking is a perfect exercise to protect your heart. The injury rate is low, and it's enjoyable and convenient. You can do it throughout the year and share the activity with a friend. And these are the very elements necessary to sticking to an exercise program for life.

Exercise Recharges Your Heart

Some of the best evidence of the heart-protecting power of exercise like walking comes from a pair of studies done by Lars G. Ekelund, M.D., Ph.D., an associate professor of medicine at the University of North Carolina at Chapel Hill. In one study, Dr. Ekelund and his colleagues put 3,106 healthy men between the ages of 30 and 69 through a treadmill test. Each man was assigned a fitness rating based on his heart rate during exercise and the length of time he was able to stay on the treadmill. Over the next 8½ years, 45 of those men died from cardiovascular disease. After adjusting for other risk factors—age, smoking, cholesterol, and blood pressure—the researchers confirmed that a low level of fitness is itself a major independent factor for heart attack and stroke.

Inactive women are also at risk.   Dr. Ekelund's second fitness study investigated women's risks.

The second study was similar to the first: 2,802 women (ages 30 to 69) were followed for 10½ years; 40 died of heart disease. Once again, a lower level of treadmill-tested fitness was associated with greatly increased risk of death independent of other risk factors, such as diabetes, high blood pressure, and smoking.

These studies led researchers to conclude this startling fact: If you don't get any exercise, your chances of having a heart attack are more than tripled.

Couch potatoes have the same risk as smokers.   The Chapel Hill researchers point out that an inactive person's risk of heart disease is the same as that of someone who smokes a pack of cigarettes a day or someone with a 300-plus cholesterol level.

An easy way to reverse wear and tear.   Extrapolating from his data, Dr. Ekelund explains that not exercising is like tacking many years of wear and tear on the heart! In effect, it ages you. But a simple program of aerobic-type exercise—such as walking for about 30 minutes three times a week—can reclaim those lost years.

Walking Tunes Up Your Ticker Six Ways

There are several ways that walking can revitalize your heart.

The most direct is by exercising the heart itself, which is a muscle. Walking gradually strengthens the heart muscle, so your heart pumps less and can rest more between beats.

In other words, walking on a regular basis helps your heart become a robust pumping machine. You decrease the number of times your heart beats while pumping more blood with each beat. All this means that you can exert yourself without feeling pooped. You can bound up the stairs, for example, without feeling like you're climbing Mount Everest.

What's more, an aerobic-type exercise like walking helps cells use oxygen more efficiently, which is crucial for people with cardiovascular diseases whose impaired circulation may cut back the oxygen supply to important organs like the heart.

Unclogs arteries.   Walking also helps prevent blood platelets from clumping together and clogging arteries, a process that can lead to a stroke or heart attack. Researchers in Finland studying a group of men between the ages of 30 and 49 found that the blood of those who jogged slowly or walked briskly for 45 to 60 minutes five times a week had less tendency to clot. The scientists speculate that the mild-intensity exercise lowers levels of a blood component that causes clotting. Just as important, they note that these beneficial effects continued for a week after the men stopped exercising.

Raises the good cholesterol.   The evidence continues to mount that walking raises levels of HDLs, or high-density lipoproteins, the blood fats thought to protect against heart disease. HDLs help cart off the excess cholesterol and fat that can clog up your arteries and set you up for a heart attack or stroke. Researchers at the University of Minnesota found that HDL levels rose significantly in obese young men who walked briskly for 90 minutes, five days a week, for 16 weeks.

"There's strong evidence that aerobic-type exercise, such as walking, does indeed raise HDL levels," says cardiologist James Rippe, M.D., director of the exercise physiology laboratory at the University of Massachusetts Medical Center and medical director of the Rockport Walking Institute.

You don't have to work up a sweat.   Even extremely moderate walking, at a pace too slow to provide other cardiovascular benefits of a brisk walk, can raise HDL levels. In a University of Pittsburgh School of Medicine study, 30 sedentary men exercised at three different levels of intensity for 20 minutes at a time. HDL levels rose just as sharply during low-intensity sessions. Which goes to show that you don't have to get your heart pounding like a piston before your body experiences a positive change.

Lowers blood pressure.   High blood pressure can lead to heart attacks. Here's why. When the blood consistently flows in high throttle, arteries become weak and narrow. When that happens, the blood supply to the heart may be shut off.

But an exercise like walking, studies show, can force the blood vessels to open up (vasodilate), and that makes the blood pressure come down and the arteries remain wide open.

In studies linking exercise with blood pressure, James Hagberg, Ph.D., a researcher at the National Institute on Aging, found that exercisers had an average 20-point drop in their systolic blood pressure (the top reading) and a 10-point drop in their diastolic (the bottom reading) after completing an exercise program. That could make a big difference to someone with borderline high blood pressure!

You may be able to say goodbye to medication.
Doctors at the University of Florida, Gainesville, Hypertension Clinic have found that walking controls blood pressure better than drugs in some people. They also report that patients with slight to moderate hypertension often see their blood pressure return to normal a few weeks after they start walking.

But even if you still need medication, you may be able to lower your dosage once you start walking on a regular basis.

Regular walking is an ideal exercise for hypertensives because unlike, say, a spirited game of one-on-one basketball, walking won't raise already-high blood pressure to dangerous levels. Yet walking gives the cardiovascular system a great workout, promoting greater efficiency and lowering blood pressure.

Also, since weight gain often triggers high blood pressure, the gradual loss of weight through a regular walking program is an additional way to bring blood pressure down.

Encourages weight loss.   Trimming excess pounds can be beneficial to your heart even if you don't have high blood pressure. The reason? Added poundage puts a strain on the heart muscle— it has to work harder to pump more blood into a bigger body. What's more, any extra calories the body has that it doesn't need turn into triglycerides—body fat. Walking can help you burn off the body fat, peel off the pounds, and ease the burden on your heart.

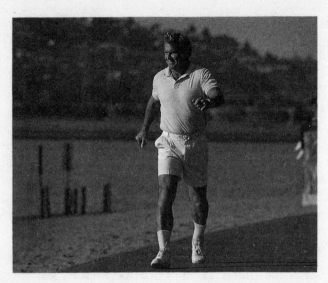

Bold new evidence confirms that walking tunes up your heart several ways: It conditions your heart muscle, helps cells take up more oxygen, clears the arteries, reduces blood pressure, and encourages weight loss, thus easing the burden on your heart.

Stepping up to Heart Health

The usual walking prescription for heart health is a minimum of 20 minutes of brisk walking at least three times per week. It's even better if you can walk every day.

But before you lace up your walking shoes and go bounding out the front door, you'd be wise to take the following precautions.

Get the go-ahead from your doctor.   Getting medical clearance from your doctor is important for veteran benchwarmers before beginning any exercise program. But checking with your physician is particularly crucial if you have a heart condition. The American Heart Association agrees that many heart patients can benefit from walking, as long as they have their doctor's go-ahead.

Your physician will probably ask you to take a stress test to detect any heart blockages and to determine how long you can walk without overburdening your heart. You will be advised of a safe target pulse rate for your exercise.

Even if you're subject to angina attacks—chest pains associated with heart disease—you may be able to safely begin a walking program. But it must be done under a doctor's supervision, in a medically supervised setting, if possible, especially if you take medication.

Advise your doctor of your medications.   If you're taking any antihypertensive medication, talk with your doctor before beginning a walking program. There are many different types of blood pressure medications, so find out from your physician the particular side effects or warning signs to watch for in your case. What's more, some hypertension medications have been shown to block the cardiovascular effects of a workout, and your doctor may advise you to switch to another drug that is more compatible with exercise. Don't change the dosage of any medicines without your doctor's approval.

Avoid hand weights if you have angina.   If you have a history of angina, don't walk with hand weights and don't carry anything weighing more than a few ounces on long fitness walks. Any added strain on the upper extremities can trigger chest pain. Also, avoid walking in very cold weather, especially if it's windy.

Forgo hand weights if you have high blood pressure.   Exercising your leg muscles won't raise your blood pressure significantly during exercise. But additional exercise of the smaller muscles in your arms can raise your blood pressure, sometimes to dangerous levels. The rule? Walk without weights.

Stop if you feel chest pain.   If you have chest pain when walking, *stop*—call your doctor immediately. Don't continue your walking program until you've discussed the pain with him or her. (If you've been prescribed nitroglycerin, make sure you always carry it with you.)

Once you have the nod from your physician, there are still a few rules to follow as you begin your walk. Though you may think that walking is a snap (after all, you've been doing it since you were a tyke)—walking for *fitness* requires a conditioning period.

Go out for a weekend of five-mile walks without proper conditioning, and Monday morning is apt to find you with painfully sore calves, thighs, or hips—not to mention blisters. So begin gradually so your body can become nicely attuned to walking and will happily carry you for regular fitness-promoting walks. Here are a few more tips to follow. (For more specific pointers on how to start a walking program, see chapter 5.)

- Wear comfortable shoes—ones that feel great, not just okay.
- Start with a stroll and work up to a stride. For the first month, your aim is to gradually work up to walking 30 minutes a day—which is generally what is needed to pump that fitness factor into your system.
- The first day, walk no more than about 15 minutes. The next day, walk just one minute more. Add an additional minute on to your walk each day until you can walk for a half hour and feel refreshed, not fatigued or sore. If you feel any part of your body straining, cut down on the amount of time you walk.
- Always walk at a pace that permits you to carry on a conversation.
- Try to walk every day. If you must skip a day or two because of foul weather, that's okay, but always aim for seven days a week. If you manage to tack 5 minutes a week onto your daily regimen, you'll be up to 35 minutes per day in just one month.
- The second month, try to lengthen your walking time from 35 minutes a day to 45 minutes. You may want to walk just a little faster. You may even want to try out some mole-size hills. But always keep three watchwords in mind: gradual, steady, comfortable.
- The investment you've made in daily walking will pay big dividends—a healthier heart and a longer life. Keep it up.

Other Body Benefits

The benefits of walking don't stop at a healthier heart. Hippocrates didn't call walking "man's best medicine" for nothing. Research shows that a regular walking program can benefit the body from head to toe. Here are some other reasons to keep in step.

Benefits for the head. You're no dummy to make walking your fitness activity, because research shows walking can stimulate thought by increasing the brain's supply of oxygen and boost spirits through the release of natural, mood-elevating brain chemicals called endorphins. Walking helps your head in other ways, too.

- It reduces risk of stroke by keeping the blood flowing freely and by keeping the arteries of the brain elastic.
- It forestalls senility by keeping blood vessels in the brain free of blood-blocking plaque.
- It reduces the discomfort of headaches by increasing circulation to both the brain and scalp.

Benefits for the bones. Bones need exercise, too. They respond to weight-bearing exercises (such as walking) by taking on more calcium and becoming thicker, stronger, and more resistant to osteoporosis—a weakening of the bones associated with aging.

Just ask Marilyn Sousa about boosting bone health through walking. Even as a young woman, Sousa saw the effects of osteoporosis. Her mother wore an old-fashioned brace to support her weakened spine. At the time, no one knew that the immobilizing corset would make her spine weaker.

Today, decades later, Marilyn has osteoporosis, too. But instead of cutting down on the action, she has stepped hers up. She walks two miles every morning and two more every night.

She has been a patient at the Osteoporosis Center at the University of Connecticut Health Center for 15 years. There, doctors make exercise an important part of a program that includes hormone or fluoride treatment and calcium supplementation.

Thanks to the program at the Osteoporosis Center, Marilyn Sousa has been able to maintain her bone mass for 15 years now. Unlike her mother, who was bound in a corset, she is bounding with energy.

Bone loss is slowed. People with severe osteoporosis aren't going to build up their bones overnight. But for postmenopausal women who are at high risk, walking may be a good way to prevent (or at least slow down) bone demineralization. In one small year-long study from the USDA Human Nutrition Research Lab at Tufts University, nine postmenopausal women walked for 45 minutes a day, four days per week. (For eight months of the study, the women wore eight-pound waist weights while walking.) After a year, they showed a 3 percent increase in low-spine bone density.

Three percent may not sound like much, but over the years it adds up. Inactive women of the same age range, who acted as experimental controls, had a 10 percent loss in bone density during the same period. The rules to follow for improving bone health:

- Keep a slow-to-moderate pace. Walking quickly could put you at greater risk for a fall . . . and a fracture.
- Be careful where you walk to avoid falling. Hills, choppy pavement, gravel, and any other uneven surface can trip you up. Slippery surfaces and dark areas are also hazardous. Curtail solitary outdoor winter strolls and night walking. (Two good places to go for a walk: an indoor track and a mall.) Take along whatever support you need to keep your balance, such as a cane or a walker. Or try the buddy system. Leaning on a friend is fine (as long as the friend doesn't mind).
- Wear a pair of good walking shoes. Look for plenty of cushion in the heel to minimize jarring and stress. The shoes should be comfortable, and you should feel like you can easily keep your balance in them.

Benefits for the lungs.   Walking might not make you huff and puff, but it's still pumping up your lung power. Studies show that a regular walking program can:

- Increase VO-2 max (the ability of the cardiorespiratory system to use oxygen)
- Strengthen muscles of the diaphragm
- Reduce the desire to smoke (now *there's* something to walk a mile for)
- Reduce symptoms of chronic emphysema and bronchitis.

A breath of fresh air for asthmatics.   It's not unusual for out-of-shape asthmatics to have attacks during physical exertion, say experts. When they start to breathe heavily their bronchial tubes go into spasms. Then they really have to fight for their breath. But, by conditioning the lungs—through gradually increasing activity—bronchial tubes become less reactive. This allows people with asthma to be physically active.

If you are still not convinced about how walking can give a lift to your lungs, consider the case of Leon Lewis. A double bout of asthma and emphysema left Lewis so breathless he had to arrange his life to accommodate his lungs. The 63-year-old New York publicist would take the bus so he wouldn't have to climb the subway stairs. He'd hail a cab rather than a walk a few blocks. He knew his four-pack-a-day cigarette habit was a big part of the problem. But he couldn't quit. He kept smoking even after severe asthma attacks landed him in the hospital—four times! His doctor warned him his next attack could be his last.

On a friend's suggestion, he started walking. "Just a block or two at first," says Lewis. "But slowly I was able to walk farther and farther. I began to see that smoking interfered with the 'exercise high' that I got when I walked. I really enjoyed walking, so I stopped smoking."

Soon after that, Lewis enrolled in an exercise training program for asthmatics at the Pulmonary Function Laboratory at New York University Medical Center. There, guided by director Francois Haas, Ph.D., he began walking 15-minute miles on a treadmill and doing other exercises while his breathing was monitored. His asthma attacks decreased. "For the first time in years, I felt like I could breathe freely!" Lewis exclaimed.

Benefits for the back.   Many runners suffer from low back pain because of the stress to spinal disks created by running's pounding. Walking, however, puts no more stress on spinal disks than standing (and considerably less stress than sitting), and it actually may help relieve back pain by strengthening and toning muscles that make the spine more stable.

"Walking affects the spine in positive ways," says E.C. Frederick, Ph.D., of the Penn State Center for Locomotion Studies, and coauthor of *Walk On, a Tool Kit for Building Your Own*

Walking Fitness Program. "It strengthens muscles in the pelvis and lower back, which may help some people with back problems."

Help indeed. An informal poll of 492 people with a variety of back problems, published in 1985, shows that "walking was helpful in the long run for 98 percent of survey participants who make it a regular part of their routine." Many of those polled said they believe walking makes their backs stronger and more flexible and improves overall muscle tone.

Walking at least two miles a day was one of the 25 most-often-mentioned ways of easing back pain. The respondents also noted that walking at least 30 minutes a day, four times a week, greatly reduces stress, a major contributing factor to back pain.

Benefits for the legs.
Walking is a step in the right direction not only for more attractive legs but also for healthier ones. Walking can:

- Slim down heavy legs
- Build up skinny legs
- Discourage the onset (as well as progression) of varicose veins.

Benefits for the feet.
For the same reason that walking is kind to the back, it's kind to the feet. Walking:

- Subjects feet to forces no greater than standing
- Strengthens muscles and tendons in the feet, so they may hurt less often.

A Diabetic's Guide to Safe Walking

Watching Walter Stein lead a pack of robust racewalkers toward the finish line, you'd have to be moved. Not long ago, the Monmouth County, New Jersey, Democratic committeeman collapsed in his office, falling into a diabetic coma. Back then, Stein was a self-confessed couch potato, crushing the springs at 290 pounds. His doctor laid it on the line: Keep it up, he told him, and you won't be around much longer.

"I knew I had to do something. But what?" Stein recalls. "Then I just happened to see an advertisement for a one-mile fun walk at the New Jersey Waterfront Marathon. Even though I'd never before in my life done anything like that, I walked it."

He finished the walk huffing and puffing. A few walks later he was hooked. Within three months he entered his first official racewalk, a two-miler in New York's Central Park. By that time he had lost 50 pounds and his blood sugar began to drop. Soon after that his doctor, Barton Nassberg, M.D., took him off all medication.

"I see a big improvement in all my diabetic patients who walk," says Dr. Nassberg. "I encourage them to walk after dinner, when blood sugar peaks. Exercising when blood sugar is low can cause dizziness in diabetics. Exercising after dinner won't have that effect. In fact, it can actually help normalize blood sugar."

His advice is right on target. Walking (with your doctor's okay) comes highly recommended by the American Diabetes Association.

How Fitness Fights Diabetes

While there are two types of diabetes, both are basically the same condition: an excess of sugar, in the form of glucose, in the blood.

Type I diabetes, which is the rarest type and is thought to be genetic, occurs when the pancreas fails to produce adequate amounts of a hormone called insulin. Insulin's job is to see that glucose gets absorbed by cells. In Type II diabetes, however (often called maturity-onset diabetes, because it's most commonly contracted later in life), the pancreas produces enough insulin—and sometimes even too much—but the insulin doesn't do its job.

In other words, for some reason the body becomes oblivious to the fact that the insulin is present. The person's cells do not respond to it. They literally become insulin resistant.

Type II diabetes is a "double defeat," according to Aaron Vinick, M.D., professor of internal medicine and surgery at the University of Michigan and chairman of the Nutrition Task Force of the American Diabetes Association. "The person fails to produce insulin in sufficient amounts, and the insulin that is produced is ineffective."

The good news is that it's possible to control your blood sugar level—and thereby control diabetes—simply by making some lifestyle changes. Along with maintaining a proper diet, exercise is one of the crucial ways to control diabetes.

Exercise enhances the effectiveness of insulin. For starters, when you move your arms and legs, you help regulate blood sugar by tinkering with insulin sensitivity.

"Exercise appears to help muscle cells take up and use sugar, even when there are lower levels of insulin in the blood," explains Gerald Reaven, M.D., a Stanford University professor of medicine and endocrinologist.

There is some evidence that exercise increases the number of receptors on the outer surface of cells, enabling more glucose to get inside the cells and provide energy. In fact, studies indicate that, to a person with diabetes, exercise acts like a dose of insulin.

Vijay R. Soman, M.D., and his colleagues at Yale University studied the effects of physical training on six healthy but sedentary men. They exercised four times a week for six weeks. After the six weeks, Dr. Soman found that the men's average "sugar uptake by insulin" was 30 percent higher—in other words, their ability to regulate blood sugar was greatly improved. He also tested each person's fitness level and found that the fitter the man, the less he showed a tendency to develop diabetes.

Even with the rarer forms of diabetes, the Type I (insulin-dependent) diabetics find that with regular, moderate exercise they can reduce the amount of insulin they need. Studies have shown that some marathon runners with Type I diabetes, for example, needed just half their usual number of units of injected insulin on the day of a big race.

It helps pounds disappear.   Exercise is important for yet another reason: It helps fight flab. Seventy to 90 percent of the people with Type II diabetes are overweight. People who are overweight seem to put out an excess of insulin, an excess which in time can numb cells so that blood sugar isn't absorbed. So the end result is the same as not enough insulin: too much glucose in the blood. Regular exercise can boost a sluggish metabolism to burn off more calories. That's why regular exercise can help people lose weight more easily and, just as important, keep it off.

It combats clotting.   Exercise can also be a boon for diabetics because it helps keep the platelets from sticking together. Platelets are tiny disk-shaped clotting elements in the blood that are supposed to bunch together when you cut yourself. Problems start when they jump the gun, sticking together when there's no cut. In diabetics, that abnormal clotting can cause problems like diabetic retinopathy, tiny hemorrhages in the eyes that can lead to blindness.

A little exercise goes a long way.   Studies have shown that lowered glucose levels and increased insulin sensitivity result from just three half-hour workout sessions a week. Researchers at the University of Vermont College of Medicine, in Burlington, put 18 overweight diabetics on a limited-calorie diet for three months. Nine of them did aerobics just three times a week in addition to dieting. Yet that single difference was enough to improve their insulin sensitivity much more than the group who did not exercise.

Other researchers found that even keeping 15 to 30 pounds off improved the patients' blood glucose levels significantly. The loss also enabled some people to decrease medication.

Why Walking is the Best Rx

"Most diabetic people know that their life span depends upon controlling their blood sugar, and also their weight and blood pressure," says Henry Dolger, M.D., former chief of the Diabetes Department at Mount Sinai Medical Center in New York City. "Exercise is an excellent adjunct to caring for all three, and the best exercise for people with diabetes is brisk walking."

The exercise doctors recommend most.   Walking is the activity most often recommended by doctors who treat diabetes. Why? Because the average Type II diabetic is 56 years old, overweight, and has been sedentary most of his life. Walking is the gentlest, most convenient way for him to ease into activity and keep it up.

Not only does walking deliver all of the fitness benefits described above but it's easy on the body and there is very little risk of serious injury.

"It's by far the safest, least stressful, and most productive of all exercises. It improves the efficiency of every unit of insulin taken in or produced by the body," Dr. Dolger explains. "That means you get more effectiveness out of every gram of food you eat than you would without exercise. It also gives you a great sense of well-being and requires no equipment." And, again, walking is a great weight-loss tool. If you walk a mile a day, burning 100 calories, in a year you'd shed more than 10 pounds which could be enough to make a difference in your blood sugar levels.

Walking clears the bloodstream steadily.   An even-paced, continuous exercise like walking helps steadily increase the demand for glucose, helping to clear excess sugar from the bloodstream.

On the other hand, an activity that's significantly more vigorous than walking could clear too much sugar from the bloodstream too quickly, leading to attacks of hypoglycemia (low blood sugar).

What's more, heavy exercise may even aggravate poorly controlled diabetes, where glucose levels are too high and insulin levels are too low. What happens then is that the liver releases high amounts of glucose into the bloodstream and the low levels of insulin can't move the excess glucose into the cells.

So don't sweat it if you have diabetes. Start strolling, and in time you may notice considerable improvement.

Check with Your Doctor

Not all diabetics will benefit from exercise, doctors caution. If your diabetes isn't under control or you have complications, exercise can make it worse. And if you have high blood pressure, that needs to be controlled first. Your doctor may want you to take a stress test, and he'll want to judge the effects of any medication you're taking.

Get the necessary exams.   If your blood sugar control is good, you should still be checked for peripheral vascular disease (PVD) and nerve damage in your feet and legs. People over 30 or those who've been diabetic for more than 15 years may need to have an electrocardiogram/treadmill test to check for early heart disease.

Have an ophthalmologic exam to determine if you have retinopathy, a disease of the retina which can be a complication of certain forms of diabetes. If present, this condition can get worse when pressure in the eye increases, which may happen during exertion. If you've got retinopathy, you may have to take extra precautions to preserve your sight.

Keep your physician informed.   After you get your doctor's approval, keep him informed of your fitness progress. As you exercise more and perhaps lose weight, your medication needs may change. But only your physician can determine that.

Exercises you should avoid.   Don't lift weights or perform any other activity that involves pushing or pulling heavy objects. It raises your blood sugar levels and blood pressure and can worsen diabetic eye disease.

Control Diabetes Step by Step

Once you get the go-ahead from your doctor, you are ready to start your walking program. Basically, you'll want to keep these rules in mind.

Aim for high frequency.   At least three times a week is good advice for the diabetic. Exercise seems to have a beneficial effect on blood sugar for up to 48 hours, so exercising faithfully at least every other day will produce the best results. Diabetics get greater benefits from several low-intensity walks per day. So rather than going on one hour-long walk daily, try two or three 20- to 30-minute walks every day or every other day.

Walk more if you're overweight.   Non-insulin-dependent diabetics, 90 percent of whom are overweight, may do well to walk five to seven times a week. This may improve the rate of weight loss.

Maintain an easy pace.   If you do skip a workout or two, don't try to make it up by walking faster or twice as far. As we mentioned before, vigorous exercise can cause a rise in blood sugar, especially in people who have an insulin deficiency.

Exercise at the same time each day.   Walking at the same time each day—whether early in the morning, over the lunch hour, or after work—helps you develop a habit of regularity. Also, the timing of exercise can help control blood sugar levels.

You may need to exercise _before_ meals.   Non-insulin-dependent diabetics may benefit from exercising before meals. This helps regulate appetite and promote weight loss.

Others should exercise an hour *after* meals.   On the other hand, insulin-dependent diabetics should not exercise on an empty stomach when blood sugar is low. They should plan their walks for an hour or so after a meal, Dr. Dolger explains, when blood sugar levels are reaching their peak.

The reason for this is that exercise can sometimes lower blood sugar levels too much, causing hypoglycemia. But if you exercise about an hour or so after meals, when levels of blood sugar are peaking, hypoglycemia is less likely.

Carry glucose tablets.   To counter a possible episode of hypoglycemia during a walk, people taking insulin should carry a few glucose tablets. They're better than a candy bar because they are more readily absorbable. Most pharmacies stock them, and they're available without a doctor's prescription. But to be safe, be sure and ask your doctor about how much exercise you can tolerate before you need to replenish your store of carbohydrates.

Drink fruit juice.   Dehydration can cause blood sugar problems, so it's wise to drink fluids shortly before walking, especially on hot days. Milk or natural fruit juices may be better choices than water because they provide you with a little extra energy for the exercise period ahead.

Avoid temperature extremes.   If the weather is too hot (over 80°F with humidity above 70 percent) or too cold (below freezing, taking into account the wind chill), for comfort's sake, head for the nearest shopping mall. Many doctors recommend that their patients walk in these temperature-controlled environments. And many malls now welcome walkers with special programs.

Always carry identification.   Use a tiny, strap-on wrist wallet or a fanny pack or a small pouch that attaches to the instep of your walking shoe to carry your vital statistics. Include your name, the name of your doctor, the names and dosages of medications you're currently using, your address and telephone number, and pertinent information about your medical condition.

The Importance of Pampering Your Feet

"People with diabetes often suffer from premature hardening of the arteries, which causes poor circulation and nerve insensitivity in their feet," says Marc A. Brenner, D.P.M., director of the Institute of Diabetic Foot Research.

Nerve damage from diabetes lessens the sensation of pain, so diabetics may not even know they've injured their feet. What's more, blood vessel damage means injuries and infections don't heal like they should—a little sore can become gangrenous, leading to amputation. Here's how to keep your feet doing what they should—walking for fitness.

Select only the best-fitting shoes.   If you have diabetes, seek out a professional shoe fitter. Make sure your walking shoe is snug but not tight, with plenty of room for your toes to move around. A shoe that has a removable insole is a good choice for those who need to insert their own specially designed orthotics (molded shoe inserts). If in doubt, consult your podiatrist.

Go for cushioning.   Today's running and walking shoes do a super job at cushioning tender diabetic feet. (A study on running shoes showed they do a better job than street shoes at preventing blisters in diabetics. Some doctors tell their diabetics to wear nothing but running shoes.)

Look for good air flow.   Shoes with mesh vents provide the air circulation that will keep your feet dry and help prevent problems like blisters and infections.

Don't forget the socks.   Wear socks with thick, cushioned heels and toes. Skip the all-cotton brands. They bunch up when wet and can cause blisters. Socks made of wool, synthetic fibers, or cotton/synthetic blends are better. They provide warmth and wick moisture away from the feet, and they prevent blisters, too.

Be meticulous about foot care.   It's crucial to keep your feet clean, dry, and infection-free. Here are some important pointers:

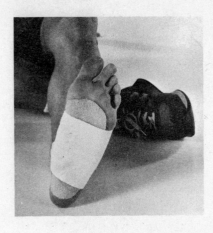

Doctors often advise people with diabetes to take up walking to control weight and regulate blood sugar levels. But diabetics who walk should inspect their feet daily. If you note any cuts, calluses, bruises, or blisters, see your doctor.

- Wash your feet well every day using a mild soap. Pat dry, and sprinkle foot powder between your toes.
- Cut your toenails short and straight across.
- Apply moisturizing lotion routinely to prevent skin cracking.
- Let someone inspect your feet daily for injuries, redness, bruises, cuts, blisters, cracks, hot spots, swelling, or infection.
- Check your shoes and socks for any foreign particles and rough spots. Change your socks during the day.
- If you develop any cracks, cuts, punctures, sores, or bruises on your feet, don't treat them yourself. See your doctor immediately. Untreated irritations could lead to infection, and infection raises blood glucose levels. If your feet become infected, your doctor should determine whether you need extra insulin.
- Have your doctor treat what appear to be simple corns or calluses, too. Don't cut them yourself, and avoid over-the-counter chemical treatments.
- Keep your feet warm on cold days. But don't use a hot-water bottle or heating pad because they can burn you without your knowing it. Don't soak your feet for prolonged periods.
- Never go barefoot.

Step Away from Stress

New Jersey advertising executive Robert Milo remembers staring for two days at a prescription for tranquilizers his doctor had given him. "I was under a lot of stress, but I was afraid of the addictive power of pills," he says. "I never did take one." Instead he saw psychologist William Rosenblatt, Ed.D., at the Biofeedback and Stress Management Center in Morristown, New Jersey. There, he says, "I found the best tranquilizer ever—walking."

He pops a special relaxation tape into his portable tape deck and heads out the door. "When I'm walking, listening to music, I can feel the tension draining from my upper back and neck," he says.

"Stress triggers your body to produce adrenaline, which readies you for action," Dr. Rosenblatt explains. "If you don't take action, though, adrenaline can accumulate, causing muscle tension and feelings of anxiety."

Walking is a positive way to move you into action. It uses up adrenaline and causes the release of calming brain chemicals called endorphins. It helps reduce tension and anxiety.

Walking also gives people a sense of control, Dr. Rosenblatt says. "When people exercise, they see that they can control (indeed, reverse) their physical reactions to stress—even if they can't control the stressful situation. As a result, they can cope better emotionally."

Work was a major headache for Robert Milo. Now his hectic day is cushioned by morning, lunchtime, and sometimes evening walks. "I'm a lot happier than I used to be!" he claims. His long laugh after that last comment lets you know he means it.

Milo is not alone in using walking as a tool for stress management and for an overall psychological boost. In one survey, over 78 percent of participants said that walking improved their attitude and sense of well-being.

While the reasons for an improved sense of well-being are complex and vary greatly according to the individual, research has shown that there are definite physiological changes that take place while you walk. And it's these changes that can help you feel cool, calm, and collected even while living in the midst of a sometimes chaotic world.

Walking: A Natural Tranquilizer

Walking can soothe jangled nerves, as evidenced in one study from the University of Southern California. There, researchers asked for volunteers who considered themselves extremely nervous.

Different means of relaxation were compared: a tranquilizer, a placebo or sugar pill (as a control), 15 minutes of walking at a heart rate of 100 beats per minute, and 15 minutes of walking at a heart rate of 120 beats per minute.

The test subjects found walking to be the best tranquilizer. Electrical activity in their muscles, which occurs with any normal activity but intensifies when tension rises, declined 20 to 25 percent after walking at both the lower and higher heart rates. This led researchers to conclude that walking is more effective and safer than tranquilizers, "and you don't have to worry about how it may interact with other medication you may be taking for medical problems," notes Herbert deVries, Ph.D., of the school's physiology of exercise laboratory.

Stroll to clear the cobwebs.   Creative potential can also be tapped through walking. "A brisk, sustained pace of about a mile every 15 minutes improves fitness levels, increases heart rate, and gets more oxygen into the blood—all of which improves your clarity. And when there's less confusion and you can think more clearly, you tend to be more creative," says Joan Gondola, Ph.D., an exercise physiologist and psychologist at Baruch College in New York City.

How to Ramble for Greater Relaxation

While you may have used walking as an opportunity to mull over problems, experts say you're better off leaving your concerns at home if you're trying to counteract stress. Instead, enjoy your walk and give your mind a rest.

How do you leave those problems behind when you step out the door? That's where meditation techniques come to the rescue. The beneficial effects of meditation as a stress reducer and immune-system booster have been well documented. Adding some meditation techniques to your walk may take you another step away from the negative effects of stress. While there are no scientifically controlled studies examining the combined activity of meditation and walking, many stress-reduction specialists feel it's a winning combination.

David and Deena Balboa, New York City psychotherapists and codirectors of the Walking Center, suggest these simple steps for enhancing the stress-reducing value of walking:

- Release yourself from any goal or objective. This is not a fitness walk with a target-heart-rate goal. Walk somewhere where you can maintain a sustained rhythm without interruption—a track or long, peaceful pathway without breaks or crossways.
- Consciously relax your shoulders. Keep your head erect to avoid contracting the windpipe and shortening your breath.
- Lower your eyelids. That will decrease the amount of external visual stimuli.

- Allow your arms their full range of motion. You will naturally begin breathing more deeply, which automatically releases tension.
- Take a few really deep breaths. When exhaling, allow yourself to sigh gently but audibly to release tension and emotion.
- Become aware of the swing of your arms and how you move your feet.
- Periodically check your shoulders to make sure they're dropped and relaxed.

Pay attention to your breathing.   George Bowman, Zen teacher at the Cambridge Zen Center, in Massachusetts, adds that focusing on your breathing and your body while you're walking brings you to a state of ''mindfulness''—a mind that's open and aware in the moment, free from regrets of the past or anxieties about the future. ''Pay attention to the rise and fall of the feet, of the breathing, until you reach a place where the mind quiets. Until, in the most fundamental sense, you're just walking.''

Walking:
The Best Antidote for the Blues

''We've found that as fitness levels increase, there are positive personality and mood changes,'' says Dr. deVries.

''We're still not sure why all this happens, but the popular theory is that it's tied to increases in adrenaline or endorphins—brain chemicals that seem to produce a feeling of well-being.

''We do know that the better your fitness levels, the greater your self-image and self-esteem. With women especially, we've found that as their fitness levels improve, they become more extroverted and have more friends. Of course, the fact that this kind of exercise helps clear up depression, anxiety, and tension is also a factor.

''Exercising gives people a sense of gaining control, of mastering their bodies and making them feel better about themselves. That feeling may then spread from exercise to other areas of their lives.''

Granted, there's a lot about depression that's controversial. And we're not suggesting self-prescribing a brisk walk for serious or prolonged depression. But if you suffer occasional mild depression, then experts suggest that a positive step you can take is into your walking shoes and out the door. Every day.

Here are some tips gathered from researchers and mental-health professionals to help you walk away from the blues.

Think ahead.   To get motivated, it may help to think about how much better you'll feel by the time you get back from a good walk.

Take some deep, slow breaths.   Do this before you start out, to begin relaxing body and mind. Once you get moving, your breathing will deepen naturally. Walk briskly, but don't push too hard. You don't want to complicate matters by injuring yourself or becoming overly sore or stiff.

Act upbeat.   Smile, lift your head, straighten your back, and imagine how you walk when you're feeling most lively and confident. Behavioral therapists say that sometimes—as simplistic as it may sound—acting happy can make you feel happy.

Plan a specific route and stick to it.   If you're feeling confused and depressed, wandering aimlessly may add to your anxiety.

Walk to the music.   If you have a portable cassette player, pop in a favorite tape. Experience the mood-altering potential of music.

Make noise.   You may be depressed because you're harboring unexpressed anger. Walking can help dissipate some of that stored-up emotion. And you can help it along by what psychologists call ''venting.'' Allow yourself a little growl or groan as you walk. Or a sigh, if you're feeling more sad than mad.

Banish tension.   Be aware of your shoulders as you walk. When you're tense or anxious, you may hold your shoulders high and create tension in your upper back. Let your arms swing, but don't force them.

Share the load.   Find a compassionate walking partner. Sometimes you just need somebody to talk to. Someone who knows how to listen without judging or giving advice. You may need to speak out about what's bothering you, instead of letting it rattle around in your head.

Walking for Peak Performance

You may already know that walking is a great way to help you unwind and keep your mood on an even keel. But did you know that a good, bracing walk can also help you rev up and set your course for the day so you can sail into daily challenges clear-headed, recharged, and rarin' to go? Indeed, a walk in the morning sets you up for the day and helps you be on time for that 9 o'clock meeting, while a brisk midday walk can help discharge pent-up tension and energize you for the evening ahead.

Stephen Kiesling and E.C. Frederick, Ph.D., the authors of *Walk On, a Tool Kit for Building Your Own Walking Fitness Program,* and David and Deena Balboa of the New York City Walking Center offer several suggestions for making your walks the perfect pick-me-up.

Set your alarm for 7:00 A.M.   That's the best time of day for a performance walk, say Kiesling and Frederick. Especially if you need to be at your best right at the start of the workday. The reason has to do with your body's temperature cycles. Your body is at its lowest temperature—and alertness—at 4:00 A.M. and doesn't normally reach its peak until evening. An early-morning walk can boost your body's temperature to the max to coincide with that early-morning meeting.

Gear up gradually.   Don't expect to jump out of bed and get right into fighting mode. Your walk can serve as your bridge into the day, both physically and mentally. Start out at a stroll, and let your body warm up to a striding pace. Stay focused on the rhythm of walking and the feeling of physical well-being that emerges from the exercise.

Clear your mind for the day ahead.   ''A common

mistake is to mentally project yourself into the future and become anxious as you imagine yourself meeting the challenges ahead. A more successful approach is to just let your thoughts dissolve," say the Balboas. "When you're involved in an activity that you have complete mastery over, like walking, you feel good, and confidence comes naturally. Maybe you won't have total control in that 9 o'clock meeting, but you will be able to rebound better because you've put your body and mind in the best condition to withstand the stress of the meeting."

Take a midafternoon perk-up.   Even if you started your day with a brisk walk, by late afternoon you may be running out of steam. The workday demands that you hold in feelings and ideas, unable to do and say the things you would like to. That buildup makes the afternoon peak anxiety time according to the authors of *Walk On*. But you can use the same walking weapon you did in the morning to defuse your anxiety and free yourself to enjoy the evening ahead.

"If you're feeling tense, you don't want to push too hard," say Kiesling and Frederick. "A maximum effort may actually increase your anxiety. But you should reach your target heart rate."

Pay attention to technique.   You can get the most from your afternoon performance walk by following these tips:

- Drop your shoulders. Late-afternoon anxiety will leave knots of tightness between your shoulder blades. Don't force them down, though. "Imagine you're carrying 1-pound weights in each hand," say the Balboas, "to gently pull down and stretch out the shoulders."
- Deepen your breathing. By late afternoon your breathing will have become shallow. Try breathing from the belly.
- Don't look down; look ahead. Find a point ahead of you so your eyes keep traveling ahead of your body. When you look down as you walk, your bent neck inhibits your breathing and keeps your shoulders tight.
- If you feel as if you're being overstimulated by your surroundings, keep your head up and just drop your

eyelids. Reducing visual stimuli will help ease your tension.

- Let your arms swing naturally to counterbalance your stride. But don't pump your arms—pumping only increases the tightness in your body.
- When you step out, let it start from the hip, not the thigh. Let your hips roll loosely to keep the hip area from tensing and to avoid goose-stepping.
- Be conscious of the rhythm of walking. If the memory of an irate phone caller bursts in on your peace and quiet, refocus on what your body is doing and imagine yourself walking through the difficulty and walk away from it.

Walk Together through Tension

Walking can help you feel good about yourself, but shared with someone, a side-by-side stroll can help you feel good about your relationship. If, for example, you're having trouble finding quiet time to communicate with a special person in your life, scheduling walking time together could solve that problem—and give both of you the benefits of exercise to boot.

Cynthia Strowbridge, a New York City psychotherapist, encourages clients to walk together, especially if they've been experiencing tension in the relationship.

"The tension can be dispersed through the exercise, rather than channeled into an outburst of emotion," says Strowbridge. "And walking together can often ease communication in another way. It's natural to have silent pauses while you walk. Those same pauses in a more sedentary setting can be awkward and anxiety producing."

Walking is sometimes better than talking. We tend to think of communicating strictly in terms of talking. But have you ever walked in silence with someone close to you and felt a strong sense of connection?

"We forget how intimate it is to be wholeheartedly with another person in silence," says Strowbridge. "Being in step

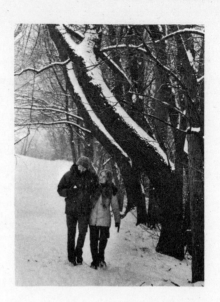

Walking with your spouse can be a special time to discuss plans and sort out problems away from daily routines and annoying disturbances. When you walk, experts say, tension is channeled into exercise and not into angry outbursts.

together out-of-doors can be amazingly healing to body and spirit.''

Strolling through understanding. It may be easier to experience this silent connectedness while walking because, in part, going for a walk together gets you away from distractions like TV, telephones, and household demands.

Jerilyn Ross, M.A., associate director of the Roundhouse Square Psychiatric Center and president of the Phobia Society of America, feels even more strongly about walking to enhance relationships since she started her nightly jaunts with her brother.

''We were having trouble getting together to just talk. We're both night owls, so after his family is in bed and my work is done, he walks to my house (about 1 ½ miles), we walk back to his house, and he drives me home. We talk and get exercise too.

''Couples, family members, and close friends have so little time to be together without disruptions,'' says Ross. ''Setting aside time to be together without distraction enhances your sense of commitment to each other.''

On Your Mark. Get Set. Walk!

by Mark Bricklin

The most important thing about designing your own walking program is to give your body all the time it needs to adapt to the special stresses of fitness walking before you push too far and find yourself hurt and discouraged.

No, I take that back. The most important thing of all is to say to yourself: I am a walker! Because only with that step, and that commitment, will you be able to carry through with the steady effort it takes to condition your body and mind to thrive on a rich regimen of walking.

Here are more safe and sane ways to design your walking program so you get more health benefits per mile.

Gearing Up

First, get yourself shod. Look for shoes specifically designed for walking. Although some running shoes will do fine, many are too flimsy, being designed more for speed than comfort and support over the long haul. Be prepared to try on everything until you find shoes that feel great.

Most walking shoes are somewhere between good and wonderful, but the key factor is how they feel on your feet. Some of us will feel good only in sturdy, thick-soled shoes, while others delight in shoes that seem nearly weightless. Some brands seem to accommodate the narrow foot best; others, the wider foot.

Now, here's the important part. Lace on the shoes and go striding through the mall. Keep moving. (For more tips for choosing walking shoes, see chapter 6.)

Good socks are important, too.   Look for socks made especially for walkers that have padding around the ball and heel of the foot. Be sure to bring these socks along when you are buying new walking shoes.

Dress in loose, comfortable clothing.   Plan to dress in layers, which can be removed and replaced as you warm up and cool down. Here are a few more tips for good walking gear:

- On cold or windy days, always wear gloves. Gloves are more important for walkers than for runners. Although runners move faster than most (but not all) walkers, they tend not to swing their arms as much. Walkers swing (or even pump) their arms energetically in wide arcs that create a surprising amount of localized windchill. This motion can numb ungloved hands.
- Wear a brimmed hat while walking in bright sunlight. Why age your face while rejuvenating your body?
- Wear a coat of petroleum jelly on your thighs—especially if your thighs are of generous cut. I was advised by a coach to grease up before a particularly soggy walk because wet clothing can produce bad chafing.
- Carry adhesive bandages like Band-Aids with you at all times, and apply at the first hint of blisters.

Plan Your Walking Schedule

The first thing you have to do is get yourself medically checked out, which I recommend to everyone. If you're over 40 and haven't been exercising regularly or if you have any health problems, medical guidance is crucial—and not just to get your doctor's okay. He or she may be able to help you in your program by recommending special precautions or tips to deal with challenges such as respiratory allergies, varicose veins, bunions, or arthritis conditions. Ask your doctor what you should look out for, both in your reactions and the elements—precautions to take in a cold wind, for instance. Many people find that their doctor's hearty approval of their intention to become a walker adds to their motivation.

Begin at a snail's pace.   The slower you progress in mileage (and speed, if you're inclined to to keep track of it), the faster and more surely you will build strength and stamina. Read that sentence again. What I'm saying is that too much too soon is the fast track to injury, fatigue, even mental burnout. You'll be walking for years, remember, so why try to hit your limits in 30 days? By taking it easy, your limits will actually disappear before you, and your progress will continue for a long, long time.

Realize that walking is real exercise.   You may think you have been doing it all your life, but fitness walking is a skill that you need to develop. If you tried to go out today and walk briskly for half an hour, you'd probably end up regretting it for the next week. Your muscles would call out indignantly that what you haven't used you have now abused. In the first month or so you're going to have all this mental energy and enthusiasm that you're quite literally going to have to sit on. If you go too fast or too far too soon, you will take longer to reach your goal of regular, energetic walking. Why? Because you'll get stiff and sore, and you'll have to rest and recuperate. And if you do that too often, you'll get frustrated and probably quit.

Aim for regularity.   Plan to walk at least three times a week and no more than six. The reason for the three-day minimim is that any less than that won't give you any conditioning effect. If too many days go by, then you are always starting over, not building strength. And though moderate walks done every single day may not hurt you, experience suggests that occasional rest days are regenerative to both body and mind. If rest days are built into your plan, you don't have to feel guilty about missing a few days here and there.

Except in the case of illness or injury, try never to let more than a week go by without walking at all. Cardiovascular improvement is never permanent! That's why a lifelong exercise program is the only answer for a longer, healthier life.

Be gentle with yourself but consistent.   Walking at the same time every day can be helpful. But if your schedule is too unpredictable for that or if your personality balks at routine, just promise yourself that sometime that day you'll fit a walk in. Don't do brisk walking before bedtime—it'll energize you, not put you to sleep.

Walk the distance that's right for you.   The "right" distance and speed are a function of your own individual capacity. And that capacity changes sometimes from day to day, often from month to month, and sometimes not at all for a decade or more. Strictly speaking, there is no minimum mileage or time at all.

A person recuperating from an illness, a person with physical problems like tender knees or 50 pounds of extra weight, a person who hasn't exercised at all in ten years, or a person 70 years of age may well be gaining significant benefits from any walking at all, for any distance. Maybe a turn or two around the block, at a speed of 1 mile in 30 minutes. Another person, fit and conditioned to long, high-energy walks, will gain some benefit from a few miles at 15 minutes per mile. And still more people benefit from greater effort—say, 4 miles at 12 minutes to the mile. But even that speed wouldn't challenge a fit, youngish speedwalker or racewalker, who may have to put in 4 or 5 miles at a fast 10-minute-per-mile pace just to get the feeling that he or she has worked out. Yet each person will have gotten a similar degree of relative improvement.

Your goal is to feel terrific, not tired.   As far as how fast and how far should you go, keep this goal in mind. You want to feel invigorated and relaxed, not fatigued or sore. Again, for some people that may mean a half-hour walk covering a mile and a half. For others, it's a 15-minute walk covering a quarter mile.

For some of you it's going to mean walking to the end of the drive-way and back. If you feel winded or out of breath, slow down or stop. Don't be concerned with keeping a steady pace at first. Right now you're just letting your body know you have some new plans for it. Keep in mind that what goes out, must come back.

Don't walk so far that you can't return easily.   Don't walk so far that you can't get back all the way around the block. Walk to the end of the street and back. If you're not sure how far you can go, keep walking around the block until you have a better idea. That way you'll never be too far from home. Remember, if you're exercising more than you were before, you're getting health benefits, no matter what the speed or distance.

Walk no faster than you can talk.   You should walk fast enough to hurry your breathing slightly but not so rapidly that you can't carry on a conversation.

Keep a walking log.   Get used to jotting down your walks: how long, how far, how you felt, where you walked. You won't be able to pretend to yourself that you're doing a good job if you're really walking only one day a week.

A Walking Guide for Beginners

Once you have mentally made a commitment to walking you are ready to take the next real steps for your walking program. But, again, don't rush into it. The first day you'll want to aim to walk a distance that is less than what you think you can comfortably cover. It may be two blocks, ½ mile, maybe as much as 2 miles, but no more. Remember to walk at a pace that barely gets your pulse up, that causes rapid breathing and no detectable muscle strain.

What you're doing, really, is saying to your body what you've already said to yourself: I am a walker! But you're not shouting it. Just making a quiet statement to your feet, ankles, shins, calves, thighs, hamstrings, buttocks, lower back, and even your arms that they now have a new job: serious walking. It will take all these structures a longer time to adapt to walking than it will your circulatory system. Later on, maybe in a month or two, you can regulate the intensity of your walk by gauging your breath, your pulse, and your sense of fatigue. But not now! If you do, you may well find that although your heart and lungs got a nice little workout, your shins or rear end or some other part of your body has been horribly abused.

And there's the tricky part. You probably won't feel that abuse while you're walking. It will hit you 12 hours or maybe 24 hours later. Just when you wanted to take another walk, you discover you can hardly make it to the front door. For some reason, the biofeedback phenomenon just doesn't work right at this very early stage, so you must strictly limit yourself to avoid nasty surprises.

Bottom line: If you want to get fit by walking, you must first get fit to walk.

With that in mind, follow this sensible guide.

Get a slow start.   First day, easy does it. Second and third days, ditto. Same distance, same speed. Meanwhile, begin to think about a steady, rhythmic pace.

Always be conscious of your body.   Are you hunched over? Are your hands in your pockets or stiff at your sides? Do you tend to lean to the left or the right? Relax and hold your head up high. Let your arms swing freely at your sides. Take some deep breaths and relax your shoulders. Studies have shown that people can affect their mood by their posture. If you look "down," chances are you're feeling down. But by consciously changing how you hold your body, there is a sort of natural biofeedback that says, "Hey, if I'm standing up straight and holding my head high, then I must be feeling good."

There is no right or wrong way for the beginner to walk except by noting what feels comfortable and what doesn't.

Let your arms swing like pendulums.   You'll find that swinging your arms gives you good balance, momentum, and a better overall workout. You may also find that your hands swell, due to the blood being forced to your fingertips. It's perfectly natural, but if it bothers you, keep your arms bent at the elbow.

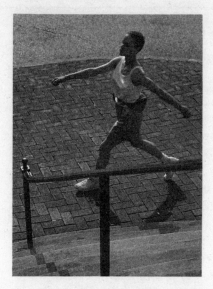

For optimum balance and a better walking workout, let your arms swing freely like pendulums. Take a few deep breaths and let your shoulders drop. Hold you head high. If your body looks "uplifted," your mood will soar.

Extend your walking time.   After walking three to five days at whatever pace you have found to be comfortable, try adding an extra 5 minutes to your walk. If that feels okay, great. Keep it there for a week or so. If not, drop back to your original distance for another week. Continue adding a few minutes to your walk until you're walking for at least half an hour, three days a week. At all times let your comfort dictate your speed. You should always be able to carry on a conversation without gasping for breath.

Step up your stride.   When you're up to 30-minute daily walks, you might want to try walking with a little more energy. Maybe covering the same distance 30 seconds faster. See how it feels. Does it seem natural? Is the good rhythm still there? Do your legs feel like they want to go at the new pace? Good!

If not, and if you feel any sense of strain or discomfort, drop back to your regular pace. Not because you can't handle the faster pace but because the slower one is right for you. At least, right for you now. Later, it might be too slow. Maybe even too fast. No matter. Remember: The right distance and pace are the ones that leave you invigorated and relaxed. Not bored or rammy, not wasted and worried. Kind of like a partner, a mate that's just right for you.

(continued on page 53)

Five Ways to Shape Up
Your Walking Form

If you've been walking for a few months, or a few years, and you feel like putting a little more zip into your walking workout, you may want to try the following tips. They are geared toward helping you get more out of a walk: more speed, more power, more stamina, more relaxation.

1.   Find your proper stride length.   If you try to go faster by taking exaggerated steps, say experts, you tire too quickly. "It is much better to take more steps using your natural stride than to take fewer exaggerated strides," says Anne Kashiwa, director of the Rockport Walk Leader Program and coauthor of *Fitness Walking for Women.* "If you step too far out, you'll actually begin to lean backward. You're trying to travel in one direction but leaning in the opposite direction."

To find your proper stride length, stand, lean forward at the ankle (like a ski jumper in midair), let yourself fall forward, and catch yourself by extending one leg. That's your natural stride length.

2.   Bend your arms.   "The long, extended arm is one thing that impedes a walker from going faster," says Casey Meyers, author of *Aerobic Walking* and lecturer at the Aerobic Center in Dallas. Partially bend your arms, crossing your body slightly in front on the forward swing, with your hand moving not higher than the top of your breast. On the back swing, your hand should move back no farther than the center of your hip.

3.   Relax your upper body.   When you hunch your shoulders in an effort to go faster, you get tension across your chest, your shoulders, and the back of your neck.

That's counterproductive to the relaxing effect walking can bring to you. And it doesn't make you go faster! Remind yourself to drop those shoulders until it's second nature.

4. Become more flexible around the hips and torso. Experts recommend that you straighten your knees so that the body rides on the bone, not the muscle. This pushes the leg up into the hip socket and promotes flexibility in the hip area. "Pointing your feet straight ahead and landing your feet directly in front of each other (like walking a tightrope) helps rotate the hips horizontally around the spinal column, another area where people are rigid," suggests Bob Carlson, championship racewalker and coauthor of *Healthwalk*. "Doing 'windmills' (rotating the arms backward, like doing the backstroke) helps create flexibility in the upper body. Stretching exercises for the hips and waist can help, too."

5. Use the psoas for more muscle power. "To walk with more power and better balance and posture, imagine that your legs begin 2 inches above your navel," say David and Deena Balboa, coauthors of *Walk for Life* and codirectors of the Walking Center of New York City. In a sense, they do. The psoas muscles, located just below the rib cage, attach to the lower spine, the pelvis, and the femur bone in the thigh and are like a bridge between your upper and lower body. By sensing that the action of your legs really begins with the psoas, you'll develop a fluid, gliding walking style—more like skating along than lifting the leg and trudging. Let your hips swing freely. You'll feel a more powerful stride because you'll be using more muscle power.

Head for the hills.   After about six or eight weeks of regular walking, you might want to experiment with some gentle inclines. No big hills, just gentle upgrades. Go a bit slower; take smaller steps and maybe deeper breaths. The exertion shouldn't be much greater than what you're used to. But the incline will involve different parts of your muscles and add variety to your walks as well. If your pulse begins racing, forget about hills for a while. If your calves or shins burn, you're going too fast; slow down! If it feels just fine, continue on the same grades for at least a week before trying anything steeper or longer. Go for slow, steady increments. Two or three times a week should be your maximum for hill work. One of these sessions could be some enjoyable weekend hiking on a nearby mountainside.

Maintain your very own pace.   One word of warning about hiking—or, in fact, any kind of walking—with friends. If others are going faster than you are, don't try to keep up. Always go at the pace that's right for you. And that should be one that you can comfortably keep up for half an hour or more.

We mentioned before that regularity is the most important factor of all in a successful walking program. Keeping a log of your walks will help you achieve that.

Practical Tips and Reminders

There are a variety of other things you can do to assure a sensible walking program that gives you the most health benefits per mile.

- Let the first 10 minutes of your walk be your warm-up period. Don't push, stretch, or move so you have to huff and puff. After 10 minutes, you might want to try lengthening your stride just a little bit—an inch, maybe. Let yourself fall into an easy rhythm. This is a good natural way of stretching.
- Your head may be in the clouds on a walk, but every few seconds, your eyes ought to be on the ground, about 10 feet in front of you. Uneven sidewalks, holes, slippery spots, and curbs are all hazardous—more so to

you than to a runner because your feet will be skimming closer to the ground.

- Always be alert for traffic. On rural or suburban roads, drivers don't expect to encounter walkers, so be extremely defensive. Don't feel bad if you have to drive to a safe place, like a park, in order to walk in safety.
- Be mindful of the weather. Dress in layers. You can always carry your gloves if you get too warm or roll up your cap or tie your windbreaker around your waist.
- Do whatever you need to do to enjoy your walks. If you're not enjoying it, sooner or later you'll stop doing it. If you need to be alone, make sure you are. If you like company, find a partner. If you need variety, change your route. If you love flashy clothes, buy something fun for walking. You know what turns you on. Go for it!

Mark Bricklin, editor of Prevention *magazine, has been at the forefront of the walking movement. An active speedwalker, Mark instituted the Walker's World column in* Prevention *in 1986 and created the* Prevention *Walking Club to actively encourage readers to walk for their health.*

Does the Shoe Fit?

If your feet don't hurt, consider yourself an exception.

In one nationwide survey, 73 percent of the people polled said their feet hurt.

Of course, there can be many causes of sore feet. Some may even require a doctor's or podiatrist's (foot specialist's) attention. But all too often, the answer is right under our noses (or toes).

According to Charles S. Smith, a professional shoe fitter for 20 years, many problems with foot pain can be solved simply by making sure your shoes fit properly. That's especially true if you're talking about walking shoes—which, of all the shoes in your closet, tend to put on the most mileage, sometimes over pretty tough terrain.

Sure, good walking shoes are designed and built for comfort rather than fashion. They have firm heel counters, wide or flared heel bases, multiple laces, padding, cushioning, and flexibility. But all that technology is worthless if they don't fit.

So how do you determine if the walking shoe fits? Smith,

who is a member of the Professional Shoe Fitters Society and the Prescription Footwear Association, recommends that you follow some simple guidelines for buying shoes your feet will love.

Nine Steps to a Perfect Fit

You are going to be racking up a lot of miles in your walking shoes. And you want to make sure you have a pair that will go the distance and not leave you sidelined with sore feet.

To help you make the best selection, go to a shoe store where you can get the assistance of a professional shoe fitter, and preferably someone who knows something about athletic shoes and the special features of walking shoes. When you find a good fitter, take his advice—be flexible and open to new suggestions. But first, arm yourself with the following information. Then the two of you can make a great team for fitting you with a shoe that will satisfy your tastes and your need for total foot comfort.

1. Don't be "small-minded."   The most common mistake people make is buying shoes that are too small. "Too often people think their shoes fit and when their feet hurt they figure they need to see a podiatrist," says Smith. "Usually by that time they do need professional help because they've abused their feet with shoes fitted too small." Foot size changes with age, weight gain or loss, and changes in exercise patterns. Never assume that just because you've "always worn a size 8," that's the size that fits you best. (You wouldn't expect your prom dress or tuxedo to fit you forever, would you?) In fact, proper fitting is often as simple as buying a shoe one half-size larger than usual.

2. Judge a shoe by its fit, not its size.   Keep in mind, too, that not every size-8 shoe is created equal. The fit will vary considerably with style and features, even within the same brand. Always have both feet measured and use that size as a starting point. Then concentrate on fit. Again, forget the size. Ask yourself, "How does it feel?"

3. Fit your "Bigfoot."   Your feet probably differ slightly in size. Make sure you fit the larger foot. It's better to add a half insole to the front of the shoe of the smaller foot than to cram the larger foot in a too-small size, says Smith.

A shoe that's a half-size too small, even though it's only a sixteenth-of-an-inch difference, can mean pain for your foot!

4. Give your toes some space.   Pay some attention to the shape of the toe of your prospective shoes. The wider and higher the toe box, the more comfort for your foot. Don't be afraid of extra space between the tips of your toes and the end of the shoe, Smith says. If you press on the toe of the shoe and hit nothing but air space, don't worry. It does not mean the shoe is too big. You need that extra room during the motion of walking.

5. If the walking shoe "just fits," don't buy it.   Many people think that if a new shoe feels roomy it's too big. Somewhere we got the notion that a shoe should fit snugly, says Smith. Maybe it's because some styles cut for fashion, such as pumps, flats, or loafers, will fall off if they're not tight. But a walking shoe should have sufficient room to allow for adequate space when your foot flexes. Shoes fitted too small will restrict the normal function of the muscles and tendons, causing pain and cramping. Keep in mind that your foot can swell to a whole size larger when you walk, and that you'll be wearing thick socks to soak up perspiration.

6. Become well-heeled.   Contrary to popular belief, a new pair of walking shoes shouldn't hug your heels. In fact, to guarantee proper fit, there should be room enough to slide a pencil between your heel and back of the shoe, says Smith. Instead, many people test the shoe's heel fit by contracting their foot and pulling up: If their heel slips out, they think the shoe is too big. They buy a smaller size and end up with blisters. (Blisters are often caused by tight shoes, not loose ones.)

The fact of the matter is that the heel of a shoe really doesn't begin to fit until after the shoe has been flexed repeatedly. Over time, the heel will "cup," or turn in at the top, and begin to conform to the curve of your heel. Professional shoe fitters are aware of this adaptive characteristic of a shoe. That's why they bend a shoe several times when they take it out of the box. They are starting that heel-cupping process for you, not just softening up the shoe.

7. Give your shoes a dry walk-through.   Try on shoes with your walking socks. And don't just stand in front of the mirror. Get moving. Walk around the shoe store or, with permission, out on the street or hard mall floor. Pay attention to how they feel on your feet and how your legs, hips, and back feel as you take stride after stride, just as you would on a morning constitutional. Are they too stiff and cloppy? Do they let through too much street feel? Does your big toe jam against the front? Your little toe against the side? Your heel slide up and down? Replace if you want to and try again. Don't buy anything that doesn't feel like it was made just for you.

8. Don't assume that tight shoes will "break in."   Discard that idea with your corn plasters. The only thing you're breaking in with a too-small shoe is your foot. As we already noted, a shoe actually gets "shorter" as your feet swell in response to walking, not longer. Shoes can get a bit wider with use, but that can be controlled by adjusting the laces. A well-fitted shoe should feel great right from the start.

9. Don't let pride stand between you and your feet.   Lots of people, especially women, feel self-conscious about wearing large shoe sizes. They tend to blush and become self-deprecating when they have to tell someone their shoe size. Don't allow this kind of social conditioning to keep you from buying the size you really need—the size that means comfort and pain-free feet!

The Best Snow Shoes

When the weather turns cold and slushy, sneakers or regular walking shoes don't seem to be enough protection from the elements.

What do experts recommend for winter walking? "A lightweight hiking boot, Gore-Tex lined for protection from moisture, is what we most often recommend," says George Pakradoonian, owner of The Urban Hiker in New York City. You get pretty good traction from such a hiking boot, and the high top protects you from twisting an ankle as well as from snow you might have to plow through from time to time. The boot doesn't necessarily need to be insulated, because then it will be more versatile and can be used in warm weather too.

As for cold-weather sock wearing, Pakradoonian suggests a wool sock with a polypropylene liner to wick away the sweat. "When your feet perspire, the sweat freezes, and that is often what makes your feet feel cold."

Wet-weather tip. Should you find yourself slogging through a sudden snowstorm or downpour while wearing your regular walking shoes, be sure to dry them properly when you remove them. Simply stuff your shoes with wads of tissue paper. The paper will absorb interior moisture as the shoes dry and help the shoes retain their shape. Never put wet leather shoes too close to a heat source—heat can damage leather just as it damages your skin.

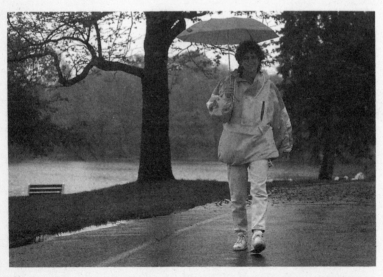

Don't skip your walk because of a few sprinkles! Wear shoes made of Gore-tex fabric that keeps wetness out but lets your feet "breathe." Ripple soles provide better traction on rain-slicked streets, and clothing in eye-popping colors helps drivers spot you through fogged-up windshields.

Good Socks Help You Beat Blisters

A good-fitting shoe is perhaps the most important piece of equipment you'll need for your fitness-walking program. But a close second is a change of socks for midwalk. Here's why. Blisters occur because excess moisture makes the skin soft, and then the abrasive action of shoe rubbing against skin is more potent.

By getting into the habit of changing into dry socks, you spare your feet from getting rubbed raw.

The best all-around socks for walking. As previously mentioned, studies show that fitted acrylic socks that allow perspiration to evaporate may be better at preventing blisters than socks made of cotton or other natural fibers. In fact, research shows that cotton socks produce twice as many blisters in runners as acrylic socks. What's more, blisters formed by cotton socks are usually three times as big as those produced by their acrylic counterparts.

"Cotton fibers actually become abrasive with repeated use, and [cotton] loses shape when wet," says sports podiatrist Douglas Richie, Jr., D.P.M., of Seal Beach, California. "The shape of a sock is critical when it's inside a shoe."

That's also why many experts suggest you avoid tube socks, those unformed heel-less wonders you can slip into without thinking.

Spun acrylic socks shape up best. For serious fitness walking, then, you're better off wearing an acrylic sock with a fitted heel. Your feet will stay comfy and dry and blister-free.

"Many people equate acrylic with a silky, nylonlike fiber," says Dr. Richie. "Yet spun acrylic feels exactly like cotton and maintains its soft, bouncy feel even when wet."

So, at the first sign of hot spots on your feet, take your shoes off, dry your feet, powder them if you can, air them, and put on your dry, acrylic socks. Be sure to wear your socks with the inseam on the outside for added comfort.

More ways to keep blisters at bay. Other ways to keep blisters from forming is to coat your feet with Vaseline or a thick ointment on your feet before your walk. This can create almost a second skin that helps protect from friction and moisture. You might also want to apply powder to your feet before putting on your socks. This can help the sock to glide over your foot a little more.

Blister Relief

If, despite taking proper precautions, you do get a blister, the best advice is to avoid letting it tear; it is better to protect a blister and let the fluid be reabsorbed.

To protect a tender unbroken blister, cut gauze or moleskin into little doughnut shapes and place it over the blister, leaving the center area open where the blister is. The surrounding moleskin will absorb most of the shock and friction of everyday activity.

The proper way to pop it.   If you need to pop a blister, use a sterilized needle and stick it in the side of the blister. Squeeze out all the fluid, but leave the skin over the blister intact. That way, the skin will eventually harden and fall off by itself, signficantly reducing your recovery time.

Keep the dressing simple.   Cover the popped blister with a Band-Aid during the day, but remove it before bedtime to help it heal overnight. Always change a wet dressing.

High-Level Fitness: What Racewalking Can Do for You

It's the darndest-looking sport. With a quick-paced waddle, racewalkers look like people trying to run with blisters on their feet.

But don't laugh. Racewalking—a featured event in the 1988 Summer Olympics—is gaining popularity among people who walk or run for fitness. And for good reason. It's a great aerobic sport that's easier on the bones and joints than running and burns more calories than regular walking. Racewalking can help you not only trim excess weight, but tone key muscles. Calves become shapelier. Upper arms, shoulders, and back muscles strengthen, improving posture. Best of all, racewalking zeros in on "problem areas"— the abdomen, thighs, hips, and buttocks. And that funny-looking hip action can whittle your waist and firm your lower torso.

So what are you waiting for? A little inspiration? Step-by-step instructions? Encouragement and support? For that and more, read on.

Confessions
of a Racewalking Convert

To an uninformed spectator, the sport of racewalking may seem like all strain and no gain. After all, if you're walking for general health and cardiovascular conditioning, speed is not important. It's consistency that counts—just walk at a comfortable pace for 30 to 40 minutes, three to four times a week. So why racewalk?

Some do it for the competition; some, to challenge their bodies to a higher level of fitness. The good news is that people of all ages can racewalk. And for those who do, the rewards are well worth the effort.

Just ask Viisha Sedlack. When she was in high school, her track coach told her she had no athletic ability. Today, at age 40-something, Sedlack is ranked number one in the world in the women's 5K (3.1 mile) racewalk.

Sedlack began running in her early thirties. She was one of half a dozen women ever invited to run in the La Rochelle Six-Day Race, considered the world championship of long-distance running. To help her train for these ultramarathon races, she turned to racewalking. In time, she found that she enjoyed racewalking more than running. So she stuck with it.

"I find racewalking more intellectually challenging than running," she explains. "You cannot let your mind drift. You must stay focused on your form in order to enhance the efficiency of the walk.

"Another advantage of racewalking is that it really improves body tone. I have trimmer thighs, buttocks, and waist than when I was a runner. And I'm impressed with the effect it has on posture—mine as well as women I've coached. Because of the vigorous arm swing, the muscles in the upper back are strengthened and the shoulders open up and straighten. People become less round-shouldered."

Sedlack counsels people on weight loss and nutrition and conducts racewalking clinics.

"My biggest thrill is to see a woman who's 50 or 60 years old compete and cross that finish line with hundreds of other athletes," she says. "One thing I've learned is that we all create boundaries for ourselves. The boundaries I break through in a six-day race are essentially the same boundaries any sedentary person breaks when they walk their first mile. People who have been sedentary all their lives start saying, 'I can do it! I can be an athlete.' "

A Beginner's Racewalking Clinic

You don't have to race to racewalk. As veteran coach Howard Jacobson says, "It's the style that counts . . . proper racewalk style promotes a high degree of fitness, even if you're not out to set records."

To reap the benefits of racewalking, you'll have to invest some time and effort to learn the technique. You'll need to focus on your body: Pay attention to your stride, your posture, your breathing. In time, says national racewalking coach Gary Westerfield, you will achieve an efficient style that will make you feel "like you're floating along . . . almost like you're dancing."

The rules of racewalking.   There are two rules for racewalking that govern technique. First, one foot must be in contact with the ground at all times. (Otherwise, technically, you'd be running.) Second, you must keep your knee straightened when it is directly under the body and over your foot. Straightening your knee automatically sends your hip jutting out.

Once you understand the two rules of racewalking, you are ready for a step-by-step lesson in the "hip" technique.

Step 1.   To get the feel of racewalking, first stand with your feet together. Relax. Now straighten one knee, allowing your hip to slide back and bend your other knee. (If you've ever carried a baby on your hip, this will feel very familiar.) Shift your weight from side to side, straightening one knee and then the other, allowing your hips to adjust by moving slightly to the side. This is the motion you want to incorporate into your walk. Try to walk around the room this way.

Step 2.   Concentrate on landing on your heel, with your

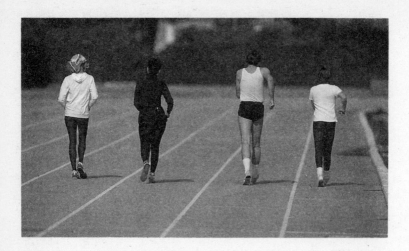

Racewalking offers important benefits: it whittles your waist, tones your tummy, and firms up your buttocks even better than regular walking. Pay attention to your stride, your posture, even your breathing, and in time, you'll achieve the perfect heel-toe, straight-leg racewalking form—an efficient style that makes you feel "like you're floating along."

foot at a 45-degree angle to the ground with your toe up and your leg straight. The idea is to roll onto your foot, making sure your knee is straightened as your body becomes centered over your leg. Having the toe up assures that your leg will be straight. Then you start to bend it as you push off with the toe of your other foot.

Step 3.   Combine steps 1 and 2. If you try walking around the room with this heel-and-toe motion, keeping your hips straight, you'll notice that you bob up and down. Instead, let your hip relax and move out as your knee straightens. You won't bounce up and down. Instead, your head will maintain an even line and you'll feel that gliding effect.

Step 4.   Move your hips from front to back, using your hip as an extension of your leg. In doing so, you can add from four to eight inches to your overall stride length. That's why someone racewalking next to you and taking the same amount of steps will seem to glide past you effortlessly.

Step 5.   Bend your arms at the elbows and let them swing from the shoulder. You'll find you can actually add momentum to your walk by pumping your arms. Just be careful to stay relaxed. A lot of people hike their shoulders up around their necks as they try to go faster.

Step 6.   Coordinate your arm swing with your stride. When your foot is forward, the arm on that side is back; when the foot is behind you, the arm is out front.

Perfecting the Technique

Racewalking takes practice. Plus all the help you can get from friends and fellow racewalkers.

According to Henry H. Laskau, three-time Olympian who won 42 National Racewalking Championships, racewalking form is difficult to master on your own. And it takes time. He estimates that it takes the average person six to eight weeks to get the technique down. Laskau advises you to learn the technique very, very slowly. Technique and form come before speed and distance, he says. Also, it's advisable to get input from a pro. If you don't know one offhand, try some of the avenues below.

- Attend a racewalking clinic where you can get feedback from experienced racewalkers. There are active race-walking clubs in almost every state. You can receive a directory by mailing a stamped, self-addressed envelope to Sal Corrallo, TAC (The Athletic Congress), P.O. Box 120, Indianapolis, IN 46206.
- Find a partner who is willing to train with you so that you can monitor each other's technique. Check each other on the angle of heel strike, for body lean (never backward and no more than 5 degrees forward), and on whether or not you're straightening your leg, says John Gray, author of *Racewalking for Fun and Fitness.*
- Read a good racewalking book, like John Gray's or Howard Jacobson's *Racewalk to Fitness,* which is generally considered the classic how-to-racewalk manual. Jacobson has years of racewalking and coaching experi-

ence. His book has a "you-can-do-it," friendly approach. Jacobson tells you how to start, how to train, how to enter races if you wish to compete, as well as how to deal with hecklers. (He's the kind of guy who likes to heckle back.) For information about the book, write to Walker's Club of America, Book Dept., Box M, Livingston Manor, NY 12758.

- Train in front of the TV with a racewalking video. And why not watch the best? Anne Kashiwa, coauthor with Dr. James Rippe of Rockport's *Fitness Walking for Women,* is also cocreator of a racewalking video entitled, *Yes! We're Walking!* by Fit Video.

    With the help of Tim Lewis, who holds the world racewalking record for the indoor mile, Kashiwa introduces the benefits of racewalking and demonstrates the techniques in a slow-motion treadmill sequence. Says Kashiwa, "You can take apart the total racewalking technique and add one motion at a time to your regular fitnesswalking workout." According to Kashiwa, the key element is practice. "You'll know when you're getting it right. You'll feel that very gliding, fluid motion. That's the reward of concentrating on this technique of walking."

Speedwalking:
Walking Fast without the Waddle

Racewalking is just one variation of stepped-up walking. After you have been walking regularly for many months, you may want a heavier-duty workout.

Mark Bricklin, editor of *Prevention* magazine, and an active speedwalker, guides you through a special five-month high-level program of speedwalking, a fast-paced walking style that can boost your fitness benefits.

Remember, though, that you don't need to embellish your T-shirt with world-class sweat stains in order to get health benefits from walking. "If it's health—and just health—you're after, remember, there's no need to walk especially fast or shed pints of sweat," reminds Bricklin. "For health, what you want is regularity of walking. You want to put in two to four miles a day, four to six days a week for a total of 10 to 20 miles a week. Twenty-five maximum. And maybe you want to walk at a pace that seems lively. Brisk . . . brisk for you. What seems brisk for me is totally irrelevant. And dangerous. Each of us has our own optimal pace. You'll know it when your walk's over, and you feel great."

If you're going for a heavier-duty workout, realize that what you're pursuing is not so much health as fitness. A challenge. Fun. All of which is perfectly legitimate, and which may be what you need to keep your walking program enjoyable.

Be sure, by the way, to get your physician's approval before you go in for gonzo walking. And check with him if you have any problems along the way.

The Secret of the Pyramid

"You begin your speedwalking program inside your head— with a mental image," Bricklin says.

He suggests that you picture yourself in a tunnel inside an Egyptian pyramid. You have just discovered an ancient cart loaded with gold jewelry and precious gemstones.

If you can manage to get that cart outside, its cargo is yours to keep. The only problem is that the wheels on the cart have grown fragile with the rust of centuries. If you push it too hard, those ancient wheels are just liable to shatter under the strain, and you will never get your treasure. So you don't push at all. What you do is lean. You lean against that cart until it begins to move ever so slowly. And you keep leaning. You don't get impatient and start shoving, no matter how slowly the cart moves, because time doesn't really matter. Only progress matters. If you get tired, you rest. Then you carry on, leaning, getting your precious cargo closer to the end of the tunnel.

"That's how you should go after advanced fitness walking," Bricklin says. "You lean into it. You don't push. You relish every inch of progress . . . you take your time. Go too fast, and the whole program can come to a grinding halt. Keep leaning into it, and success will be yours.''

With that image ever in mind, you are ready to begin your program.

The equipment you'll need.   Besides your walking shoes, you'll need just one piece of equipment: a digital sports watch. Read the instructions. Find out how to go from the time of day to the elapsed time mode, because you're going to be timing yourself.

Determine your walking course.   Find a walking course that is about one mile long or that takes you about 15 to 20 minutes to cover at your usual speed. The exact distance isn't important. Just be sure to make note of start and stop landmarks at both ends.

As for the lay of the walking course, imagine one that has uneven sidewalks, nine or ten traffic lights, steep hills, unchained pit bulls, major earth fissures, and a couple of fumaroles (volcanic craters). Got that? What you want is the exact opposite. Your best bet is a park, though a tree-lined residential area can be almost as good.

How to Time Yourself

Once you have selected a suitable walking course, you're ready to take the first steps on your actual speedwalking course.

Day 1.   On the first day, include your special fitness course on your usual walking itinerary. When you reach the starting point, start the stopwatch. Walk at your usual speed to the end of the course, then freeze your time. Make note of it. This is your base time for what we'll call Course A.

Day 2.   Go back to Course A. But before you begin walking it, warm up. A walking warm-up is very simple. All you do is walk—at a normal, easy pace for about 15 minutes. Take a couple of deep breaths along the way. Flap your arms around, rotate your shoulders, swivel your hips. That sort of thing. Vigorous stretching before walking is counterproductive. That's because the stretching will place far more strain on you than the actual walk! And done when those muscles are cold, it's even worse. If you are used to doing a stretching routine and you've never injured yourself stretching, save it for when you get home and your muscles are warm.

Having warmed up, go to your starting point, hit the right button on your watch, and begin your walking again. For the first five minutes, proceed at the same speed you did yesterday.

Pick up speed after 5 minutes. At the 5-minute mark pick up your speed. Don't do that by taking longer strides. Longer strides only strain your muscles. Just move your legs faster. A little faster. Don't pump your arms or do anything other than take faster strides. After about 4 or 5 minutes, return to your normal pace and continue to the end of your walk. Stop your watch.

Check your body. Does anything ache? Are you winded? Do you feel strange? If you feel anything other than great, you're not ready for advanced fitness walking. Carry on with your usual walking, and try again in a month. If you feel really bad, see a physician. Probably, though, you'll feel just fine.

Check your time. Note the time on your stopwatch. Ideally, you've shaved off 10 or 15 seconds from your time. If your time is the same as it was yesterday, not to worry. Tomorrow, try again. If you can take those 10 or 15 seconds off your time tomorrow, you're on your way. If you can't—at least without straining—then forget about advanced fitness walking for the time being. Resume your regular walking routine, gradually add some distance to your route, and then try again in a month. It's possible that you're already getting your personal maximum benefits from walking and trying to go faster will only distress you.

On the other hand, if your time for Day Two is more than 30 seconds faster than Day One, you're going too fast for comfort! Even if you don't feel any discomfort, you may be putting too much stress on your shins, hamstrings, groin, or buttocks. Those are the areas that need the most time to adapt to speedwalking.

Good Morning, Pulse

How does your stepped-up walking program affect your body? You are about to find out by measuring your pulse.

Day 3.   On this day, you begin taking your pulse. You must always do this early in the morning, at the same time, preferably a few minutes after awakening. If you take your pulse any later, the count will be subject to random increases by activity, worry, or eating.

Two ways to take your pulse. The first way is to place the tips of the first two fingers of your left hand on the inside of your right wrist, about half an inch from the right side. Or you may prefer to place the tip of the thumb of either hand on the tip of the chin, and then reach to the outside of the windpipe with the tips of two fingers. Just let your fingertips rest where they sense a strong pulse. Don't press, because you won't get an accurate reading.

Using your digital watch—or perhaps watching the one on the news bulletin cable channel—count the number of beats for a full 60 seconds. That number is your A.M. Resting Pulse.

Monitor your pulse. Write down your pulse on your graph, or simply remember it. More to the point, you're going to watch the downward trend of your pulse over a long period of time as a barometer of your fitness level. Sustained, vigorous exercise performed at least three times a week does that to your pulse. As your heart and other muscles become more efficient, they learn to process oxygen from the blood more efficiently, slowing your heart rate.

The average pulse rate is said to be about 72, though many are naturally higher or lower. A pulse in the low 40s or lower may sometimes be associated with cardiac problems. But speaking in very broad terms, a fit person may have a resting pulse of about 60; a very fit person, in the mid-to-low 50s. Serious aerobic types may have pulses in the 40s or even 30s. "My own pulse was 60-ish when I began jogging some years ago, and fell to 48 after a few years," says Bricklin. "When the back pain produced by running led me to take up speedwalking, my pulse stayed at that value for a few months. But as I began speedwalking for 45 mintues a day, it fell all the way to 41."

Keep in mind there is tremendous genetic variability concerning resting pulse and its response to exercise.

The more you walk, the slower your pulse. Don't expect any drop in your pulse in the first few weeks of your fitness walking program. What you're basically doing in those early stages is conditioning your body to be able to walk rapidly. Before too long, though, watch for your pulse to begin slipping downward. It's a slow process and may only become evident over many months or not at all. A drop of five or six points over a year is significant, and any more than that is truly impressive. Eventually, your resting pulse will stabilize, and your continued walking will keep it there.

A smart walker, by the way, also takes his blood pressure and gets regular medical checkups.

Clocking Your SPM

So now you're out on your walking course, and you're going to repeat yesterday. But you'll add one new trick.

As you're doing the faster portion of your walk, glance at your digital watch, and take note of how many strides you're getting per minute. Count each contact of your right foot with the ground as one stride. You will probably be cruising at about 60. One stride (actually two steps) per second. Or close to it. Whatever it is, write it down on your graph when you return home. There is nothing magical about that number. But like your pulse, it can be a valuable gauge of your progress over the long haul. Speed, remember, is not produced by unnaturally long strides but by rapid strides.

"The first few days of my fitness walking career, I averaged a perfect 60 strides, minute after minute," says Bricklin. "I remember thinking, 'It's probably impossible for me to walk any faster than this.' About six months later, I remember going for a walk in Los Angeles on a business trip and the jubilant feeling I had when I hit 75. About a year after that, I was able to cruise at 84 SPM (strides per minute). And when I speedwalked—pumping my arms and really using my hips, I could maintain a steady 92 SPM. On a short burst, I could break a hundred.

"All of which will win me no prizes, but I enjoy knowing that now I can easily perform physical feats I thought impossible years ago."

Day 4.   You're still a fledgling at this fitness-walking business, so don't try to break any records. Repeat the same routine you did yesterday. Today, though, be conscious of your posture. You should be fully erect. Your shoulders relaxed. Your arms swinging like pendulums. Look ahead of you about 15 feet, but occasionally sweep the scene to check out any foot hazards. Take a couple of deep breaths every minute. Just a couple, though. And with each breath, relax your shoulders. Make note of your time, which should be about what it was on Day Two.

Day 5.   If you wake up without any serious tenderness in your legs, you're doing well. And you're ready to resume "leaning into fitness." Increase the time you spend speedwalking along your course by about one minute—say, from four mintues to five, or five to six. Look to shave a few more seconds off your time.

Day 6.   Repeat the exploits of Day Five. But don't try to go any faster. Give your body a chance to catch up with your enthusiasm. And check your feet today. Any sore spots? Baby blisters? Take care of them now!

Day 7.   Take the day off. You can stroll, ramble, even hike, but don't do any fitness walking. In fact, always give yourself at least one day off a week. Maybe two. You need it, mentally as well as physically. The rambler can do his thing every day; the fitness walker can't and shouldn't.

Listen to Your Inner Coach

You've been striding along at increasingly greater speed for a week. For the rest of the month, you will step up your stride even further . . . but gradually, safely . . . all the while paying heed to signals from your body.

Second, third, and fourth weeks.   Every few days, explore the experience of increasing the fast part of your fitness walk by another 15 seconds. Be guided by your inner coach. Never strain. If you're grunting or gasping, if you sense your shoulders tightening, your posture bending forward, or your stride becoming uneven, back off. If you feel weak, dizzy, or strange at any time of the day, quit walking and see a doctor. The reduction in time you experience over your approximate one-mile course may slow down in the later weeks of the month. Or you may find the greatest time reductions toward the end of the period.

Shave a half minute off your time in a month. After a full month, a reduction of 30 seconds off your base time for the course is signficant. A reduction between 30 and 45 seconds is highly significant. More than 1 minute? You just got ticketed for speeding. Take it easy.

If your time hasn't decreased at all, but you feel better for the exercise and you're having fun, wonderful! Keep at it. But don't go on to the routine that follows until you can comfortably reduce your base time by 30 seconds or more.

Fifth week. Something new again! We're going to add some arm action. So far, you've been letting them swing like pendulums. Now you're going to bend them and use them like pumps to help your legs propel you.

Use the bent-arm technique. The important thing is to keep your shoulders relaxed, so that your elbows are swinging in the lowest possible arc. If your fists are flying around your upper rib cage, they're too high. Get them down to your waist.

You may recall reading about this curious arm technique in the section on racewalking. When you try it, it may feel funny at first. You may be a little self-conscious. The first runners felt self-conscious, too.

But notice what this new technique does for your time. It should be worth another few seconds, anyway. And you'll be getting valuable upper-body exercise, too.

By the end of the fifth week, the time you spend speedwalking along your course will probably be between 10 and 12 minutes. Don't forget to take your day off!

Polish Your Form

By the middle of the second month, you should be ready to concentrate on smoothing out your speedwalking form.

Sixth week. Try walking a bit more erect; use a little less or a little more arm action, whichever gives you a smoother gait. And always land on your heel, never on the midfoot or toes.

Don't hold in your stomach. Remember to relax your lower belly, and imagine your breath going all the way down. But don't suck wind like a steam engine with every step. Do that only for three breaths at a time, once a minute. Then remind yourself to keep your shoulders low and relaxed.

Seventh week.   If you're feeling good, try walking the length of Course A at a fast clip. You may have to slow down some in order to stretch out the effort. Count your SPM's during the first and last minutes of your walk. If the first minute's count is higher than the last, even out your pace. Do this check regularly in the future. Jack-rabbit starts are not a good training technique.

Eighth week.   One day this week, measure a new walking course that is either two miles long or that takes you about 30 minutes to cover when walking at a normal speed. Record your time and start-finish landmarks. This is Course B.

On your other days, continue walking the length of Course A at a rapid clip. Don't forget to record your times and graph them. (By now you're finishing your second page of one-month graphs.)

Your pace may level off. Don't feel discouraged if your times aren't getting faster. Plateaus are part of the natural landscape of fitness walking. Your body is adapting at its own sweet speed. You are better off being guided by that inner coach than by arbitrary goals of improvement.

Third month.   Alternate between Course A and Course B. Gradually lean into Course B so that each week you're quick-stepping a greater portion of the course. By month's end, you may have worked up to speedwalking the full length.

Remember to warm up by walking a normal mile before starting your timed course. Afterwards, walk normally for 10 to 15 minutes to cool off.

Make Friends with a Hill

As already mentioned in chapter 5, walking uphill is one of the best ways to add a bit more challenge to your walks.

Fourth month.   First, scout out every hill within walking distance. The ideal beginner's hill is a long, easy one that most people wouldn't complain about. If all you can find is a rather steep hill, you will have to downshift into your lowest walking gear.

Know the facts about hill walking. There are two key points about hill walking. One, walking a hill at a speed that's even a little faster than normal is surprisingly difficult. The amount of energy needed rises much faster than the apparent angle of ascent. So take it real easy. Listen to your inner coach and slow down, or even rest for a while if necessary.

Second, the muscle fibers used in walking up and down hills are slightly different from those used when walking on the level. So even when you are nicely conditioned to speedwalking a flat course, you need a fresh set of adaptations to tackle hills. Hill walking is a sure way to produce sore muscles. Give yourself plenty of time. Hill walks should only be done perhaps twice a week. And don't worry about timing yourself on hills. That could lead you to push too hard.

Set a new hill course. Your third walking course—call it Course C—should include the hill. When you do that, begin a new set of records.

You've Become a Fitness Walker!

By the fifth month, you are getting into the groove. You have your favorite route, or maybe two, and a special time of day to walk it. You're taking pleasure and pride in shaving a second here, a second there. You also know that some days you aren't going to shave anything, and even that can feel good. You've become a real fitness walker.

Keep paying attention to style. Maintain a smooth, graceful gait, landing on the heels and pumping the arms straight ahead. Have someone watch you—or catch your reflection in a big window. Does your head remain level as you walk? That's good! Are your shoulders riding higher than normal? That's bad! Do you look a little trimmer now than you did four months ago? That's great!

As you continue fitness walking, you'll shape up not only your style and your profile but also your health and your self-esteem. And because fitness walking is so much less damaging to the body than many other sports, you'll be able to go on enjoying these benefits for the rest of your life.

Keep walking!

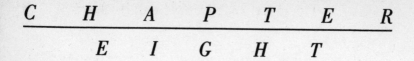
How to Keep Your Walking Program on Track

The sky is gray. There is a nip in the air. And your determination to get out and walk has faded like the leaves on the trees. Besides, your schedule is crammed today—trying to squeeze a walk in just doesn't seem worth it.

When the skies are cloudy or your schedule is crowded, it's easy to skip a day or week of walking and take solace in the belief that you'll catch up.

But a week off may stretch into a month and before you know it your walking program is gone with the wind.

With a little advance planning, you can fit a walk into a busy day and get your body in gear no matter how gloomy the weather. For suggestions, read on.

Eight Ways to Stay Motivated

Don't wait until the spirit moves you to start moving your feet. The key is to have an incentive plan handy for those days when it is extra hard to get out the door. The following list might just give you the little nudge you need.

1.   Get the big Mo working for you.   It's called momentum, and pro athletes know it can make or break a sporting contest. It can also help you get up and out on your walking route. About an hour before lacing up your walking shoes, start thinking about the walk. Imagine how good it'll feel to get outside in the fresh air and how invigorated you'll feel afterward. Reflect on the physical and emotional benefits that come with a good walk. Psyche yourself. Granted, you're not about to play the Super Bowl or World Series, but the stakes, in terms of your health and well-being, can be just as high.

2.   Get some walking literature.   Go to the library and check out books on walking. It helps to see that there's more to walking than merely strolling around your block. Pictures of people walking in all kinds of locales—from cities to suburbs to country lanes to desert roads—are good inducement because the images get you in the walking frame of mind and remind you that it's an activity for anywhere and anytime.

3.   Pretend you're walking across the country.   Keep track of your mileage, and use pins or a bright marking pen to plot your imaginary progress on a map of the state or nation. You may be intrigued to see how far your fanciful trek takes you. Think of the bragging rights: "I walked across four states this past winter," you might say.

4.   Add variety to your walking regimen.   Boredom comes easily when your routine repeats itself day after day, so vary the time of day you walk. Also establish different routes for a change of scene. If your paths are limited, at least reverse directions periodically. If weather conditions are just too harsh to be outside, head for the nearest shopping mall. The environment is controlled and predictable, and you're safe from dogs, traffic, rocks, hills, and allergy triggers like pollen.

Think about substituting a leisurely stroll in place of faster-paced striding. The aimless ramblings along wooded paths and the meanderings through parks to people-watch or feed the ducks can regenerate you and give you respite from inner turmoil. These casual saunters can stretch the spirit as well as your muscles.

5.   Set goals.   Take a "now" photograph of yourself and list your vital statistics on the back—weight, resting pulse, and blood pressure, for instance. Tack the picture where you'll be sure to see it, as a reminder that you'll be checking your vitals again in a few months and comparing the numbers. Charting your progress

The Most Important Motivational Tool

What's the key element in maintaining your walking program? Your walking log. You will find that this log contains a strange magic, a power to encourage and inspire you to go beyond even your own idea of what you expect to accomplish this year.

This is where you record your moments of truth. The first truth: You walked or did not walk. The second truth: You walked two miles or three miles or 10 minutes or an hour. The third truth: You felt lousy; you went faster; you slowed down.

If you really want to create a walking program that will give you genuine health benefits like better muscle tone, cardiovascular improvement, increased circulation, and all those other good things, *use* your walking log. Fill in all the dates so you can see the empty spaces as well as the ones where you've jotted down notes.

In a few weeks you'll begin to see the magic . . . like pride in your accomplishments and inspiration for making the day-to-day commitment. This log will talk to you and will become your impartial ally on your footpath to better health.

To create your very own walking log, get a notebook and make a few columns. In the first column, jot down is crucial because the feedback is encouraging, and you can proudly show your results to others.

6.   Remember all the calories you'll burn.   Like most people, come midwinter, you may have overindulged in holiday fare or be nibbling more because so much time is spent inside. But keep in mind what you learned from chapter 1. That is, if you walk at an easy-to-moderate pace for 40 minutes, at a rate of about

the days of the week, Monday through Sunday down the left hand side of the page. Make the next column the date. The third column is the hours or miles you walked. And the final column is for your comments. Here is where you will note your experiences, body response, weather, anything you feel is significant. Keep track of your week's total hours and distance at the bottom of the page.

Somehow there is a reassuring sense of fullness and security when you can look back to a certain day and know, "Yep, walked three miles that day around Trout Creek Park. It was drizzling and foggy but the mist off the stream was eerily beautiful. Felt relaxed and peaceful."

Don't forget to add a variety of notes to enhance your pleasure and personal awareness. How about keeping track of your daily weight, your resting pulse, your time for a mile? Even if you're not trying to break records, the results can be interesting. Another way is to add more subjective words about your mood, feelings, what you mused about on your walks. What great ideas did you spawn, what problems did you solve, what daydreams did you drift through? That may make for some exciting reading in a future quiet moment!

20 minutes to a mile, you'll have walked 2 miles. That means a 140-pound person can burn 190 calories, and walk off 5,700 calories after 30 days. Since 3,500 calories equal a pound, you've walked off a pound and a half. After six months, you'll have shed 9 pounds without restricting food intake.

7.   **Walk with someone.**   When you're absorbed in conversation, the time passes faster and you may not even notice the harsh weather. Having a walking mate also makes it harder to skip walks because a good partner probably won't let you get away with it.

In fact, studies have shown, that if you're having trouble sticking with your walking program, teaming up with a partner may help you stay motivated. Fifty-one men enrolled in a hospital-based exercise program at St. Francis Medical Center in Peoria, Illinois, were twice as likely to stick with their walking program for a year if their wives also exercised.

8.   **Join a walking club.**   As the saying goes, the more the merrier. The sense of camaraderie can help instill a desire to walk, as can the good-natured spirit of competition that comes with a group activity. Knowing that other people are out there walking in the dark days of winter can be good stimulus, too.

How to Work In Walking

Once a career-minded person has scrambled up the ladder of success, what's on the top rung? Chairs, that's what. Chairs for meetings, for airport waits, lunches, commutes, and the rest of your routine. And the higher you climb, the less often you need to get up: When you're really top brass, someone can always bring in your food, your messages, your meeting participants, your paperwork, and your chauffeur.

But all that lack of activity will eventually take its toll from your health, your energy level, and your attempt to control your weight. The more sedentary your job becomes, the more you should find ways to work in physical activity—and walking, the easiest exercise, is the activity that can fit into anyone's day. Adding more frequent walks to your daily routine is even more important

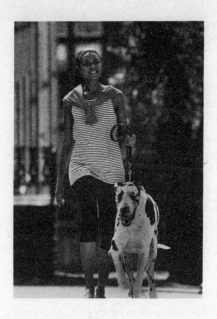

Some people have found that a four-legged companion can keep their walking program on track. After all, having a dog to take care of forces you to get out and walk every day, no matter how busy your schedule or how blustery the weather.

if you exercise infrequently or if, like many executive "weekend warriors," you save up strenuous pursuits for off-hours once a week.

Here are a few easy ways to work in walking.

On the job.   Need to talk to your assistant privately? Planning a lengthy phone chat with another department head? Invited to a lunch date or happy-hour rendezvous with a colleague? Instead of picking up the phone and leaning back in your chair, suggest a brisk walk—even out of the building—for such one-on-one discussions. You'll both feel the better for it, and you can't beat the privacy of talking as you walk, especially outdoors. What's more, the activity can ease the tension of what might be a difficult discussion and heighten the energy in a positive chat.

On lunch hours.   Start by skipping the elevator on your way out, and take the stairs as you warm up. Then if your office is in a suburban location—but not on a wide-open campus, ideal for walking—drive to the nearest enclosed mall. You can window-shop while you stride briskly around the mall a few times. If you're city-bound, figure out the longest loop you can take in a nearby park or around several long blocks. Pick up your lunch toward the end of the loop, then complete the cycle by carrying it upstairs.

On your coffee break.   Next time you need a pick-me-up, try walking around the block instead of heading for the coffee or candy machine. Walking, explain researchers at the California State University, is the pause that refreshes longer. What happens when you eat a candy bar is that your blood sugar rises, but only briefly. Within an hour, it dips again and you feel droopier than ever. A brisk ten-minute walk, however, can boost your blood sugar and energize you for as long as two hours.

Don't be surprised if, after your walk, you're struck with a great idea or two. Researchers found that walkers enjoy much greater improvement in response time, visual organization, memory, and mental flexibility than people who do not exercise. Apparently, when you pump your legs you're also pumping more oxygen into your brain cells. Perhaps that's one reason why many of the great thinkers—from philosophers like Aristotle to scientists like Albert Einstein, as well as many famous writers from Walt Whitman to Henry David Thoreau—were also avid walkers.

On your commute.   If you've ever sat in a car, bus, or train stalled by traffic and thought, "I could walk there faster"—try it! On a weekend or a less-hectic workday, find the best way to wedge walking into your commute pattern, particularly if you use public transportation. You'll avoid some of the lines and crowds and arrive energized. Get off the bus or train one stop sooner on the way to work and board one stop later on the way home. Don't forget to park your car as far from the station as possible if you take a train in; it'll force you to add more paces to your walking day and let you find parking space easily as a bonus.

As an alternative, consider commuting earlier in the morning and later at night, and use those pockets of extra time to walk when you reach your destination. A brisk stroll will allow you quiet time to recover from a particularly hectic commute in either direction, providing you with an easy way to reduce the day's stress before you arrive at your office or home.

On your corporate campus.   What better way to use all

those winding drives and wide-open spaces? If you have to meet with someone in a department located in another building, walk rather than drive. At lunchtime, spend half an hour striding along the roads (or, if you're lucky, on community walking trails). Entertaining clients on their first visit to headquarters? Take the opportunity to give them a walking tour while you discuss business.

On a daily basis, arrive slightly early so you can park in another building's lot, and walk over to yours to start the morning with an extra shot of energy.

On business trips.   When you have to see several clients in another city, try to arrange your meetings in advance so you can allow time to walk from one to the next. (The city's chamber of commerce can send you a street map to help your planning.) The benefit: You won't waste time hunting down cabs, and walking will let you reflect on your last meeting as well as rev up for the following one. Add even more walking time by taking stairs in your hotel or in high-rise buildings where the meetings are located. And if you find yourself in airports frequently, take advantage of their wide-aisled indoor protection and walk your way through the inevitable waits. (Check your luggage first or leave it with a companion.)

On errands.   Whether you do them on your lunch hour, on weekends, or when you arrive home, consider walking your errands rather than "running" them in your car. If you prefer to pick up several items in a mall or shopping center, choose distant parking spaces and walk rather than drive from one end of the center to the other.

Warm Up to Winter Walking

Don't take winter sitting down. While it's tempting to hibernate in the family den or TV room, there's nothing more invigorating than a brisk walk in the cold, crisp air.

In fact, research has shown that exercising in cold temperatures may shift the body's metabolism into high gear. So you burn more fat as your body tries to stay warm. But if you have asthma or heart or circulatory problems, consult your doctor first.

Getting fired up for frigid walking.   Start by making
the decision to walk in the wintry morning the night before. Then,
follow these suggestions to keep walking when it's cold outside:

- Lay out all your walking clothes before you go to bed.
  Think layers for more insulation. The inner layer,
  ideally, should be polypropylene to wick away perspiration. The second layer is the insulator. A wool sweater,
  for instance, helps trap body heat. The outer layer
  protects you—try a zippered windbreaker, a light shell
  that cuts the wind and wetness. Take along a wool cap
  and a scarf to pull up over your face.
- Eat some warm cereal one hour before going for a walk.
  Then drink a warm beverage right before you go out.
- Prepare your body for cold air by doing simple range-
  of-motion exercise to gently stretch each body part
  indoors first. By the time you hit that cold air, you will
  already be warmed up.
- Cover your face and lips with petroleum jelly.
- Wear sunglasses that protect against the sharp sunlight
  bouncing against snow.
- If the wind is blowing, walk against it at the beginning
  of your walk. At the end, walk with the wind and
  you'll be exerting less energy when you're tired.

How to Choose
and Use a Treadmill

Think of it! A temperature-controlled environment. No wet
leaves. No icy patches. No potholes. No snarling dogs. Just you
and your treadmill.

Once the domain of serious runners and cardiovascular physicians, treadmills have caught the interest and imagination of recre-
ational walkers. And why not! For anyone on a walk-a-day
schedule, they offer the ultimate in convenience. And they may
help you increase the effectiveness of your workout.

According to Patrick Netter, author of *High-Tech Fitness,* the
electronic or motorized treadmill motivates you to maintain a
certain pace. "If you stop walking, you fall down," says Netter. In

addition, if you want to challenge yourself to a more vigorous workout, you can simply increase the treadmill's elevation to simulate hills. With some models, you can program a warm-up and cool-down, or train at intervals that push you to your limit and then ease you back to a comfortable pace.

Set your track in front of a TV or even a full-length mirror and the time will fly while you walk.

Prices for treadmills can range from around $200 to $5,000. Generally, the more you pay, the sturdier the construction. The pricey models also boast extras, such as automatic elevation and computer capabilities, including calorie-counting and course-setting features.

Selecting the best.   But what's right for you is based on a number of important considerations, and price is just one. If you're considering the purchase of a treadmill, here are a few tips:

- Be sure to get a written warranty.
- Buy from a specialty fitness-equipment store. The salespeople are usually knowledgeable about the equipment they sell. Often, the shop will send someone to install the treadmill for you. And, if you have a question or problem later, you'll have someone to call.
- Pass up the nonmotorized versions. They are practically impossible for walkers to use effectively. The belt creates too much of a drag, and you use all your energy pushing rather than walking.
- Choose a motorized treadmill that's appropriate for your weight and walking speed. While the more economical versions are made of flimsier materials, many of them will probably stand up fine for a 150-pound female walker. A 200-plus-pound male will need sturdier stuff. Make sure the belt is wide enough for you to walk comfortably.
- Test it in the store at a minimum speed of 4 mph.
- Look for a DC (direct current) motor. AC (alternating current) motors have to work through a system of pulleys and levers to change speeds. DC motors generally run more smoothly and have more accurate settings.

The knack of walking in place.   A treadmill is a relatively simple piece of equipment. But here are a few pointers to help you adjust safely to the new experience:

- Start slowly! When getting on a treadmill, be sure to use the handrails or hand bar. Straddle the belt with both feet, then step on. Begin at a very low speed and slowly adjust to your pace.
- Give it your full attention. Don't expect to watch your favorite TV program on your first "walk." Get used to the machine first.
- Learn to be light-footed. A treadmill is for walking, not tramping. If you plod along, you may disrupt the evenness of the belt motion.
- Don't jump off. Straddle the belt, hold onto the rails, and step off—very carefully. If you've been on the treadmill for any amount of time, you may feel dizzy and unbalanced for a few moments when you get off. Just walk slowly around the room until you've adjusted your equilibrium.

This Year, Try a Walking Vacation

If wintertime makes you drag your feet through your walks, then get busy planning a walking vacation for spring or summer. Besides giving you something to look forward to, you'll have a purpose in mind: to be in the best possible shape for your upcoming warm-weather excursion.

A walking vacation offers an alternative way to really vacate your daily grind, get a fresh fix on things, see a new part of the world, and do your health a big favor.

How does it work? It's simple: Drive to some town, city, or seaside that intrigues you, park your car at the hotel, and leave it there until you're ready to come home. During the interim, get about by means of that time-tested conveyance people used to call "shank's mare": your own two feet.

An imaginative browse through the road atlas can give you some inspiration. Delightful rambles await you in places scattered all over the continental U.S. and Canada—some of them, no doubt, not far from your home. They're varied enough to suit any temperament: quaint and cobbled, like Colonial Williamsburg or Michigan's Mackinac Island (where horse-drawn carriages, bicycles, and feet are the only modes of transportation allowed on the island), or bright and bustling, like lakefront Chicago or downtown Montreal.

Six Great Walking Cities

In some cities, particularly those with historic or restored areas, the local chambers of commerce have developed walking tours that will guide you, by means of a designated guide, a map, a rented cassette tape, or even a painted line, through the most interesting parts of town. It sometimes helps to know something about the historical background of what you're seeing, but you might prefer just striking off for parts unknwown, armed with comfortable shoes, curiosity, and a map.

As writer/naturalist Joseph Wood Drutch once observed: "You learn a city by walking it."

And that marvelous sense of discovery you experience when exploring a strange city on foot makes getting fit a real joy. Here are some great cities to discover up close:

Monterey, California.   A "Path of History," marked by a painted line winding through town, leads the walker to every old house of distinction. The setting for John Steinbeck's *Cannery Row,* Monterey's calm harbor, white beach, and red-roofed white stucco houses make it a picturesque stroll.

Contact: Monterey Chamber of Commerce, P.O. Box 1770, Monterey, CA 93942, (408) 649-1770

Nantucket Island, Massachusetts.   Once the world's greatest whaling port, Nantucket (located south of Cape Cod, 30 miles at sea) has retained its seafaring flavor, though it has become a popular resort. Its whaling museum, restored lightship, lovely beaches, and period homes on cobbled Main Street make for some very charming walks.

Contact: Nantucket Island Chamber of Commerce, Nantucket, MA 02554, (508) 228-1700

Newport, Rhode Island.   You can walk in any direction and find something interesting in Newport: the tremendous mansions along Bellevue Avenue; the Touro Synagogue, the oldest synagogue in America; picturesque restored areas; the three-mile ''Cliff Walk'' overlooking the sea. Cassette tours are available.

Contact: Newport Chamber of Commerce, 10 America's Cup Avenue, Newport, RI 02840, (401) 847-1600

Quebec City, Quebec.   Considered one of the most beautiful cities in the Western Hemisphere, Quebec is built on two levels: the Upper Town, perched on a rock citadel visible from 20 miles away, and the Lower Town, spreading up the valley of the St. Charles River. The city has more than just a European flavor. Its population is nine-tenths French, though English is understood many places. The narrow steeply angled streets, lined with stone buildings and ancient trees, are perfect for walking. Cassette tours are available.

Contact: Quebec City Chamber of Commerce, 17 St. Louis, Quebec City, Quebec G1R 4R5, (418) 692-3853

Santa Fe, New Mexico.   The oldest capital in the United States and once the end of the Santa Fe Trail, this charming city is located at the base of the Sangre de Cristo Mountains, where the climate is cool and refreshing. Local highlights include the Palace of the Governors, the oldest public building in America, but just walking the old, storied streets provides the most fun.

Contact: Santa Fe Chamber of Commerce, P.O. Box 1928, Santa Fe, NM 87504, (505) 983-7317

Savannah, Georgia.   Sitting on a high bluff overlooking the Savannah River, Savannah features the largest urban historic landmark district in the country, covering over two square miles. The scene of fierce fighting during the Revolution and the Civil War, today the city's 20 parks and squares and its revitalized waterfront area make it a great walking city.

Contact: Savannah Chamber of Commerce, 301 W. Broad St. Savannah, GA 31499, (912) 233-3067